# GLAMOROUS
## BY
# *George*

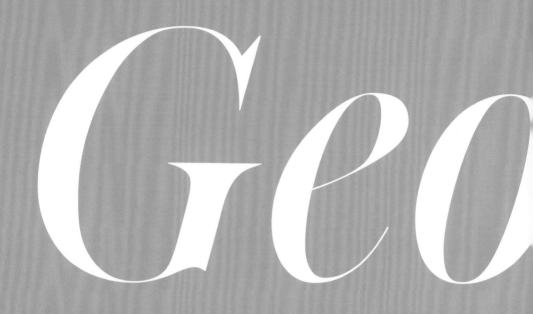

# GEORGE KOTSIOPOULOS

 THE KEY TO CREATIN

# GLAMOROUS BY

*rge*

**MOVIE-STAR STYLE**

ABRAMS IMAGE, NEW YORK

*I dedicate this book to women who take an
extra moment every day to look great,
who honor and bless all of us with their glamour.*

# CONTENTS

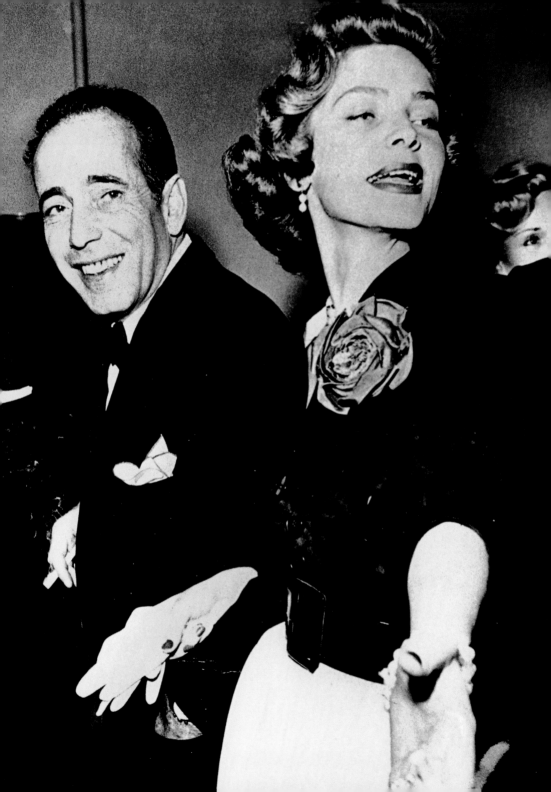

# the *glamour* of hollywood

## isn't what it used to be.

**YES, WE'VE GOT GORGEOUS CELEBRITIES** draped in couture on loan. We've got huge stars dripping with borrowed baubles from the world's most prestigious designers and jewelers. But what happened to that certain movie-star magic? The enduring qualities that made Hollywood classically glamorous are nowhere to be found on today's red carpets.

I miss iconic women. Especially today, looking out into a sea of overnight boldface names, many of whom are defined by dalliances and headline-making disasters. I long for the return of the real movie star: the allure, the wit, and the mystique.

As a stylist, red-carpet commentator, and cohost of the show *Fashion Police*, I witness the good, the bad, and the ugly on a daily basis. Growing up, I loved fashion and went shopping with my older sister constantly. I have always been fascinated by how clothes change over time, and how trends shift first on television shows and then, later, on the streets of the small town where I grew up. For instance, did you notice how differently the cast of *The Brady Bunch* was dressed at the beginning of the show, when it was prim and mod (what we would now call *Mad Men* style), than toward the end, when their clothes became much more groovy, with oversize collars and huge bell-bottoms? If you don't know what I'm talking about, DVR the show or watch a few clips online. Marcia and her siblings did a complete wardrobe change, as did *Wonder Woman* and the ladies of *Charlie's Angels* a decade later, this time from bell-bottoms to straight-leg pants.

Maybe it's just me noticing these things, but pop culture is a great place to observe fashion change. That's part of what I do on *Fashion Police,* and it's an important part of my job as a stylist. I work with celebrities, models, and ordinary women to help them look their best from head to toe.

But while I am constantly surrounded by a bevy of screen-worthy beauties and television superstars who are counted among the world's most gorgeous women, I still find myself asking: "Where have all the movie stars gone?"

Sure, I see plenty of *celebrities* during awards shows and Hollywood functions, but let's be clear: A movie star is not the same thing as a celebrity. Movie stars are of a different breed, and their staying power is absolute. In today's world, celebrities are a dime a dozen, and we count "Real Housewives" as style icons, but possessing true movie-star quality means shining brighter than anyone else in the room and commanding the right kind of attention with grace.

The world needs more movie stars, not just on-screen and at premieres but on a practical, everyday level. Just think how much more beautiful and pleasant your office, favorite bar, or local Starbucks would be if people ditched the frumpy clothes and grumpy attitudes and instead opted for elegant ensembles and charming manners on any given Thursday. This is not some pipe dream—with the advent of inexpensive but beautifully designed clothing available nationwide, elegance is within everyone's reach. And *Glamorous by George* will show you the way.

There's too much unsightly reality in the world today. Girls dressed in disheveled or skimpy ensembles have become ubiquitous. Short shorts, hooker heels, and minidresses have reached new heights, leaving little to the imagination and even less to be desired, fashion-wise. Take a character like Christina Applegate's Kelly Bundy from the 1980s–1990s show *Married, with Children*…. At the time, she was seen as trashy and extreme—a poster girl for slutty groupies, clad in a bustier top, skintight skirt, and an acid-wash denim jacket draped loosely around her shoulders. Today the Kelly Bundy look is relatively tame and would pass for something we see fourteen-year-olds sporting in the pages of a chic, glossy magazine like *Teen Vogue*. The lack of class in clothing and media may signify a shift in the way we live, but it doesn't mean that we have to abandon the magic, mystery, and glamour that give a movie star his or her timeless shine.

I would love to bring back the refined elegance of the movie star en masse. But since I can't convince the whole world all at once, I'll start with one woman at a time. Creating movie-star style may seem like a lot to do, but in *Glamorous by George* I'll show you how to look glamorous—and make it seem effortless—one chapter at a time.

As a stylist, I help clients and celebrities look great by choosing styles and fabrics that flatter their bodies and hide their flaws and by using colors that complement their complexions and personalities. I'll guide you through every step my clients take to help you find your inner movie star, from the style and color palette in your clothes to your tasteful demeanor. Luckily, presenting timeless glamour doesn't require a celebrity budget or securing a film debut at the Cannes Film Festival—just a state of mind.

You may think that movie-star style is beyond your reach, but I promise you it's not. Some of the biggest, most iconic, gorgeous, and now-established movie stars made the same leap you're about to make. When I was an assistant stylist, I worked with Charlize Theron on a shoot for *Esquire* back when she was a mere model. She was bubbly and upbeat and running around the set half naked and fully wild. She was like many other model-actresses I had worked

# LET'S GET STARTED

**We can begin your movie-star style makeover in this very introduction. Here are ten extraordinarily easy things you can do right now to bring out your inner movie star:**

★ **1.** Chic sunglasses are a movie-star must. Find a pair that's trendy, but more importantly they should perfectly suit your face shape. Take photos when you try on new shades if you must, or bring along a friend who will be honest with you about what makes you look great.

★ **2.** Stand up straight! Posture is everything. Have you ever seen a movie star slouch?

★ **3.** Be calm and pleasant to everyone, especially the nasty bullying types. It's really hard for someone to be mean to you while you're being extra nice back.

★ **4.** Be gracious, smile, and say please and thank you even in the most taxing circumstances.

★ **5.** Yes, Mama always said to wear clean underwear just in case you were in an accident, but what about wearing a cute outfit in case you become swarmed by paparazzi, accidentally walk through a TV shoot, or even worse, run into an ex or high school rival!

★ **6.** Send thank-you notes. It's not old-fashioned, but timeless, classy, and gracious.

★ **7.** Brush up on current events before a party, so you are informed and have interesting opinions to contribute.

★ **8.** Wear a little something sparkly regardless of the time of day. I said a little, don't go crazy. Pick a bracelet, a pendant, a nice ring, or even a scarf that has a touch of glitter to make your look stand out.

★ **9.** Stop saying "I would look like her too if I was a movie star with money to hire a personal trainer, stylist, chef…etc." That's just a lame excuse lazy people tell themselves. Movie stars are not lazy. YOU are now a movie star so you are not lazy.

★ **10.** Track suits and workout clothes are for the gym. Period. Replacing your favorite "running around" sweats with an actual outfit (nothing crazy, think a relaxed, yet chic striped top and great jeans) will make you carry yourself with more composure and confidence. Even wearing a chic or elegant matching set of pajamas at home instead of worn-out yoga pants will make a difference in your attitude.

with, but there was a spark to her that stuck with me. About a year later, we crossed paths again, on a photo shoot for *InStyle* magazine. This time Charlize was on the cover. She wasn't a half-naked wild child running around the set but instead a golden goddess in our midst. It was apparent through her gracious nature and the elegant way she carried herself throughout the shoot that she had made the transition from model-turned-actress/quasi-celebrity to a bona fide movie star. That day, I felt like I had witnessed an exceptional change—which ultimately led Charlize to winning an Oscar.

That transition, and its lasting impression, is what I want for you.

W HEN I'M REPORTING on red-carpet fashion, looking like a movie star is what everyone is trying to do, and hearing that they look like a star is the ultimate compliment. When people—from grannies to fashion magazine editors—use the term, it means that an actor or actress looks stunning, exudes the spirit of a screen legend, and is successfully conveying his or her own brand of modern-day iconic glamour.

But here's a big secret no one will tell you: Dressing for the red carpet and having movie-star style is easier for the average woman than for a celebrity. Think about it: Celebrities are being photographed from every angle possible, *in high definition,* whereas you can choose which angle is the best for each and every outfit you take photos of, and you just have to look gorgeous in real life. (To be entirely truthful, some of the dresses we critique on *Fashion Police* actually work in person but photograph terribly. Or the photographer has taken the worst angle on an actress possible. Or it truly is terrible.)

However, just because you're not going to be in front of paparazzi doesn't mean you can't be just as glamorous as an actress on the red carpet. I'll show you how to use the same tools of the trade that movie stars do when you're getting ready for your next date, job interview, or an average Monday. But it's important to note that channeling true movie-star style doesn't just exist on the red carpet or in looks alone. It's a collection of distinguished qualities that effortlessly

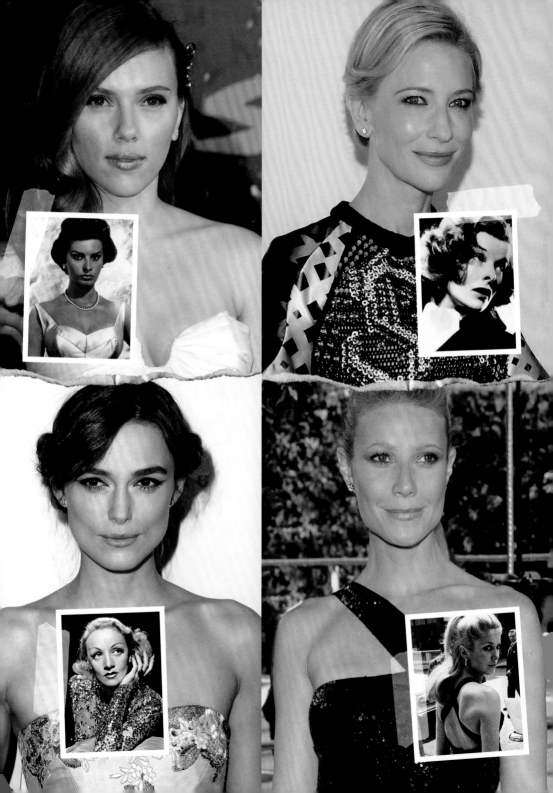

transpire in one's daily life. In *Glamorous by George* I'll show you not only how to achieve a movie-star look but also how to project the grace and timelessness all true stars share.

More so than anything else, movie stars are movie stars because of the way they carry themselves. A movie star holds his or her head high, the face is relaxed, and the overall presence is flush with confidence. *Confidence* trumps most things.

A modern-day movie star like Julia Roberts is a perfect example. I recall the first time I worked with her on a photo shoot, when I understood immediately that she possessed all the makings of a true movie star. Roberts is enigmatic, kind, and carries herself with confidence. When she smiles, you immediately know she's the real deal, and when that smile is directed at you, *you* feel like a movie star. I took a lesson from that: The truly glamorous make those around them feel glamorous and special.

So you weren't born with a naturally megawatt smile and endearingly infectious laugh? You don't have a movie-star figure? Don't sweat it! Most of us are in the same boat. A lot of women who aren't exactly prom queen material in their youth evolve to be gorgeous and glamorous on the inside and out.

When we talk about movie-star magic, we are often talking about the leading ladies of Hollywood's Golden Age, whose image and legacy still influence the way stylish people dress, fix their hair, do their makeup, and essentially walk

## RED CARPET LOOKS VS. HIGH FASHION

 There's a big difference between red-carpet style and high fashion, though certainly some actresses bring high fashion to the red carpet. One of the most fun things about working in this industry is observing and commenting on custom couture looks and high-concept fashion worn at red carpet events. (A great example of this is Lady Gaga wearing a dress made of meat.)

This is part of what we talk about on *Fashion Police*, and though I completely encourage you to keep an eye on these looks and discuss their merits with your fashion forward friends, wearing high fashion or couture clothes is not required for red-carpet style.

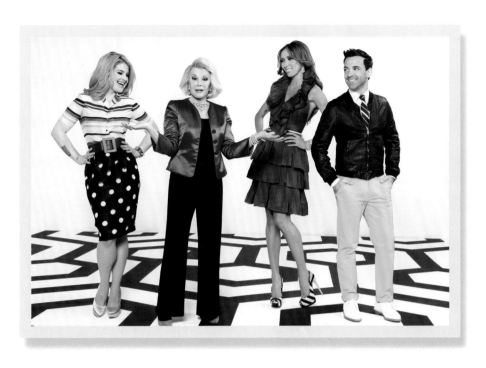

**Your hosts:** *The Fashion Police from left: Kelly Osbourne, Joan Rivers, Giuliana Ranci, and moi!*

and talk. Thus, when you look for inspiration on movie-star style, stars of that era like Katharine Hepburn, Audrey Hepburn, and Elizabeth Taylor—as well as their present-day contemporaries Emma Stone, Natalie Portman, and Angelina Jolie—are great examples of how to present timeless style and luminous presence both on-screen and off.

Part of the fun in transforming yourself is dreaming about who you want to become, or what look and image you want to present to the world. Do you want to be a bombshell, like Sophia Loren or Scarlett Johansson? Or are you more of an intellectual beauty, like Katharine Hepburn or Cate Blanchett? Perhaps you're a minimalist, like Gwyneth Paltrow or Catherine Deneuve? Or would you prefer to be more of a model-actress type who embraces trends at the edge of fashion, like Keira Knightley or Marlene Dietrich?

It's OK if you don't know which "type" you want to emulate yet, or you think you might be a cross between two different styles. (I know plenty of women with bombshell outsides who rock intellectual beauty style, as well as some who dress like model-actresses on special occasions but are minimalists most of the time.) It's also OK to be a little intimidated by the process of changing your look and aiming for movie-star style. You might be thinking, "I could never look like Emma Stone" or "How do I compare to Audrey Hepburn?" When you watch awards shows and see Angelina Jolie looking perfect, it's easy to think, "I will never be like that."

But I'm here to say you can! Not in a literal sense, of course—reading this book will not turn you into Angelina Jolie, unfortunately. But being iconic and looking like a movie star isn't just reserved for actresses. You can be your own icon—everyone can—by working with what you were born with, embracing what is best about your looks and personality.

You may not be wearing the most expensive dress, and you may not be the most famous person in the room, but you can certainly carry yourself as though you are. People will notice. Movie-star glamour begins on the inside. Let's say that again, because it bears repeating: Movie-star glamour begins on the inside. How do you go about this? Confidence is key, but so are graciousness and good behavior. You can be a low-maintenance person who doesn't fuss too much about clothes or makeup, but that doesn't mean you have to live your life without elegance. Or you can be a traditionally glamorous person on the outside, hair done, jewelry in place, and nails manicured, but let that attention to detail extend to how you treat people with grace and kindness. (Or both!)

Think of this book as the red carpet rolled out to you—helping you make glamour easy to recognize and implement in your everyday life no matter who you are, where you live, or how much money you make. ★

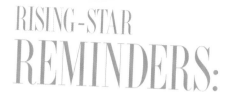

# RISING-STAR
# REMINDERS:

- ★ You can live a first-class lifestyle on a coach budget!

- ★ Movie-star style starts on the inside. Confidence gets you further than designer.

- ★ While mimicking a certain actress or era can be a great start to overhauling your look, true movie-star style is unique. Who are *you*?

Incorporating movie-star style can seem like a daunting task. To help ease your transition, I've included a list at the end of each chapter recapping its lessons. These checklists will allow you to keep reading without forgetting a single tip or trick, and they can act as reminders after your inner movie star debuts!

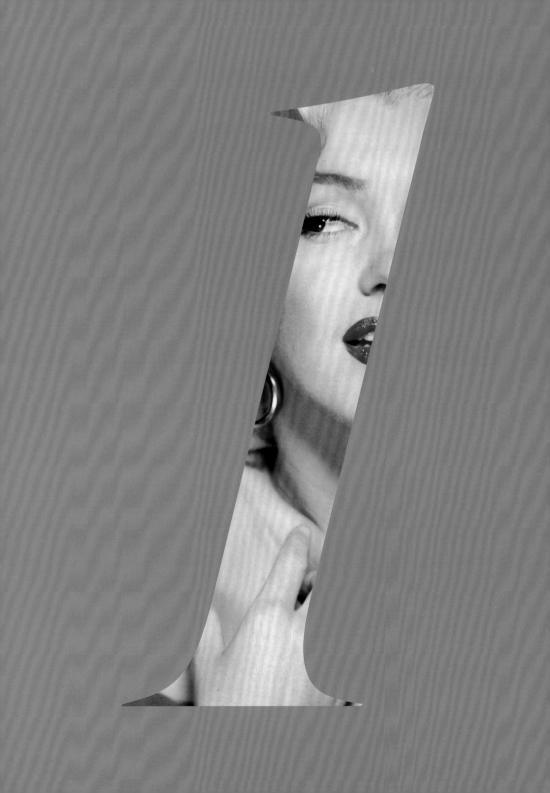

# dressing like a
# *movie star*
## *(on an extra's budget)*

T HE FIRST STEP IN CREATING MOVIE-STAR STYLE involves a costume change. Movie stars look great on the red carpet, in magazines, and even in candid photos because everything they wear flatters their natural beauty while simultaneously projecting their personality and style. In theory, your closet should do the same. I say "in theory" because that's not how most people's closets are in real life. Most people have a few things that work but more pieces that simply don't work, that are too big or too small, that don't flatter their shape or complexion, that are outdated, or that hold sentimental value and not much else. Needless to say, a movie star would not have this closet. That's why you're reading this book and coming to me for advice, because I've seen movie stars' closets. (And I have a movie-star-worthy closet myself!) A movie star has had her closet curated so that each and every piece she owns makes her look—and more important, feel—glamorous, timeless, and fabulous. But you don't have a stylist. Until now.

In this chapter, I will explain how I style my clients, and I'll teach you how to be your own stylist—a classic movie-star move! We'll not only clean out your closet but also pinpoint what's working for you now, what will work for you in the future, and what you should be shopping for from this moment forward. We'll also do your colors (that sounds so eighties, but whatever, it *works*) to figure out which shades you can wear and which you should avoid so you never appear blah again. From what hair colors work best to what shoes to keep, this chapter will help you clear your closet and build the foundation of your movie-star style.

# Color Is Black and White

WHEN IT COMES TO COLOR, camel is my enemy. Though its creamy beige-brown is a beautiful shade I like when other people wear it, wearing camel myself always makes me feel off. I feel that way because that particular shade of tan-beige-brown makes my complexion look sallow, sickly, and yellowish—ew! Most of us have a color or two that we don't like because it makes us look terrible, since only people with skin tones at the very ends of the spectrum—the palest of pale (think Anne Hathaway) and the darkest of dark (think Viola Davis)—can pull off wearing any shade of every single color on the planet. That's why I say color is black and white. Some of us (like Anne and Viola) are lucky enough to be at the ends of the spectrum and can wear anything. But most of us vary, from skin tones that are very cool (black) to very warm (white).

You probably have heard that you look great in a color, have a preference for one color over all others, or even notice an abundance of one color in your closet. And that's totally fine—if that color works for you, of course! If you wear it constantly and none of your stylish friends have stopped you, it probably does. My primary rule for color is: If you feel good in a color, and people compliment you on it—"Oh, that color is so nice on you"—then wear it. If you don't feel good in a color—for any reason—don't wear it! Simple as that.

Some people simply hate a particular color. For one of my clients, it was purple. She hated it, and even though she looked amazing in a violet sweater I begged her to try on, she refused to buy it because she hated the color so much. And though I hate to put something that fabulous back on a hanger instead of in my client's shopping bag, I had to agree. If you hate a color, you shouldn't wear it.

But keep in mind that looking bad in one shade doesn't necessarily mean you look terrible in all facets of that shade—or that you'll look horrid in it forever. It's like sushi—at first, you may not like eel, but after your palate expands a little bit more with texture, you love splitting a special roll topped with a little bit of eel. A lot of my clients (and friends) claim they don't look good in one basic color (say, red) because someone at some time in their lives didn't think a certain tone was right with their skin tone at that time. But your skin tone changes with the season (more on that coming up!), and shades alter a lot within the same color family. For instance, brick red is totally different from strawberry red. Be careful about what you think you "know," because you might be wrong. Even changing your hair color slightly can alter how you look in different shades. Next time you shop, try on a color you claim doesn't work for you—because it might work on you today, even if it didn't yesterday.

It's important to remember that even if you love a certain color, especially if you have a lot of pieces in those shades within your closet, you should make sure all of its shades work for you, either by following my rules (up next!) or by asking a friend or colleague: "Do I look good in this?" Surveying the public is always helpful, because they have a more objective perspective than you do. Shades vary a lot within color families, so a cool sky blue is different from a warm navy. So even if a friend tells you navy is a no-go, you shouldn't automatically nix the entire blue section of H&M.

It's also important to remember that just because you love a color, that doesn't mean it works for you. (Hello, camel!) After all, a lot of people love UGG boots and Crocs, both of which I'm mentioning here only because they are the

# HAIR APPARENT

## George's quick guide to cut and color

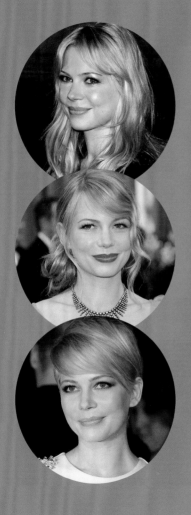

## *Length*

Long hair has become insane. With the immense popularity of extensions and weaves, I see tons of women sporting limp locks. Frankly, if your fake hair doesn't look real or is scraggly, that's not movie-star style. If your hair ends up looking lifeless long, you would be better off rocking a shorter style, like a bob or a pixie, that is equally, if not more, chic. Keep in mind hair just past your shoulders is still long hair—don't go crazy trying to "go" long, because anything past that is truly a girlish look. Thus, I advise that women should only wear their hair past chest level before the age of 35-ish because after that it tends to look tacky.

Classy looks you'll never age out of include short cuts, shoulder-length hair, and/or layered cuts no longer than your chest. It's also helpful, after 50, to lighten your hair around your face to soften the overall look.

And, lastly, if your hair cut, color, or style resembles a Real Housewife, go to a salon. Stat. No, seriously. Drop the book and go NOW!

**Great lengths:** *Michelle Williams going long in 2001, mid-length in 2006, and short in 2011.*

eBay or at a consignment store (if it's a designer piece, it probably is), whether it's in good enough condition to donate, or if a friend would like it. Some brands sell very well online, especially high-end labels like Chanel and Dolce & Gabbana, but some mid-level brands as well. It's so easy to do a quick search on therealreal.com to see what an item (or something similar) typically sells for. Let's say you have a fuchsia Yves Saint Laurent bag. Check out what similar Yves Saint Laurent bags in bright colors have sold for, in what condition, and you'll be able to gauge what you would end up getting for it by reselling.

Most of us have friends who would love a designer piece, so consider giving the clothes that don't quite work for you to either a friend or a deserving charity. Glamour is about giving, not greed.

## Figure out what's missing.

Ever have that moment when you're trying to get dressed for a day at work or a fun social outing and have no idea what to wear? Everyone does—even me! But focusing on it *when* you stand in front of your closet is key to fixing it and making it work for you like a movie-star closet would. For instance, if you're standing there drawing a blank every time you have a first date,

then you clearly need a super-cute first-date outfit! (That can be repeated until you meet The One, and then you'll have to add date-*night* outfits…) For the next week or two, make a list of every time you look into your closet thinking "ummm…" and what occasion you're trying (and failing!) to get dressed for. It can be anything: cocktail hour with the girls, an office party, or just a Wednesday before work.

One thing many of us overlook when cleaning out our closets (and when shopping) is what we may be missing from our *outfits*. Would a new scarf that highlights the colors in your wardrobe really make your blouses pop? Are you always cold, or looking for an extra layer? Perhaps a great cashmere cardigan or a leather jacket would help. Adding these components to your list will help you solve fashion dilemmas just as much as figuring out what events in your life you feel you have nothing to wear for. After all, having *something* to wear isn't the same as having something fabulous to wear!

✳ As I've mentioned before, for every fashion rule, there's an exception! It's usually Lady Gaga, but in this instance … well, it sort of is and sort of isn't. The exception in closet cleaning is formalwear. If you have a special-occasion dress you love and that looks great on you, by all means keep it—even if you haven't had a chance to wear it yet or don't wear it often. Celebrities do this all the time—and trust me, if you love that piece enough, you'll find a place to wear it.

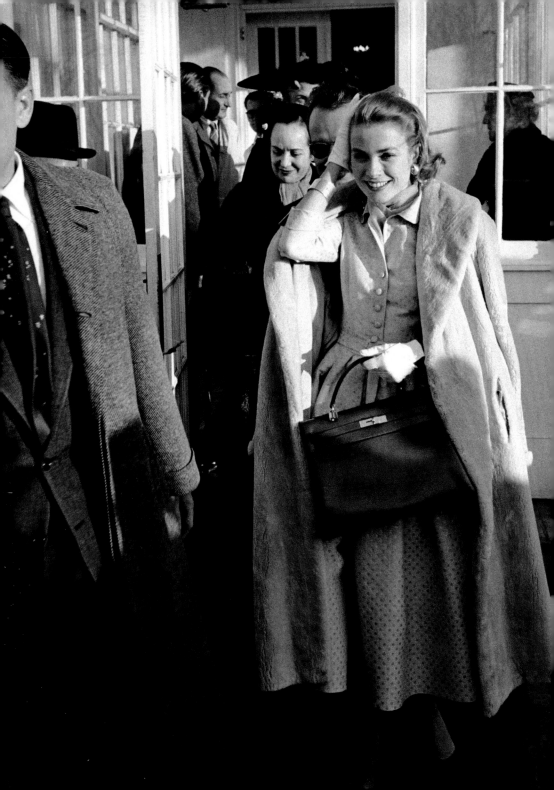

# A WORD ABOUT
# HANDBAGS

A lot of women buy expensive handbags because their favorite celebrities rocked the same bag at a great restaurant or on the street. But guess what? That celebrity didn't go buy that bag. The majority of the time, she was given it for free. While that does mean she likes the bag enough to carry it, it doesn't guarantee that it's emblematic of her style or that she would have picked that bag out herself, given the chance. It's a simple marketing scheme: Designers send free swag to celebrities, and then when celebrities are photographed with the swag, their sales go up.

Some A-listers I work with, including Oscar-winning actresses, opt out of this altogether by donating any free bags they receive to charity. True movie-star style, as these A-listers demonstrate, involves being gracious, not greedy. (But don't get me wrong—a few of these bags squeak into even the most generous A-lister's closet. Even movie stars love free stuff!)

Everyone wants to look and feel special—that's why you're reading this book! But often, buying a trendy or designer bag makes you less special, not more, because so many other women end up buying the same item. Using your newly honed knowledge about color and a sense of your own style, look for day bags that have a design and an impression in line with the image you want to present. Feel free to look at celebrities' bags for inspiration, but be brave and do your own thing.

Collect as many day bags as you'd like. When you get tired of using one, keep it if it's in good condition. It may become your go-to when you redis-cover it in your closet six months from now, or you can give it to a friend or sibling who loves it. And since you're going to elevate your style, why not shop for a classic evening bag? Black, gold, and silver are timeless and always work for movie-star occasions, even at the last minute.

# WHAT HEEL HEIGHT SHOULD YOU WEAR?

The paparazzi spot movie stars in all sorts of heels (or lack thereof) these days. But what you wear personally is a combination of height and your own style. If you're tall, you can certainly wear flats all day (and at night, for casual occasions) if you'd like. If you're short, you could wear heels all day, especially in the styles that are more comfortable to wear, such as wedges and stacked heels. If you're in between, a small stacked heel (like an oxford) can be comfortable and stylish. But only you know your day. If you're going to be in an office sitting, then a four-inch heel isn't a big deal, whereas if you are on your feet at work or running after kids all day, wearing high heels would be quite a painful—not to mention ridiculous—afternoon!

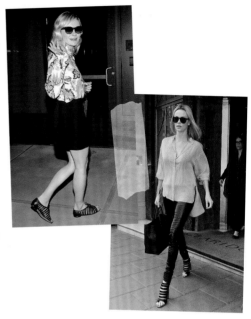

certain items in specific styles. You'll wear what works for you, no matter what's in your closet, so telling you to go buy Louboutins or a Chanel jacket isn't really going to matter if you'll never wear them.

That said, the wrong shoes can change your overall impression from starlet to star-struck. While overhauling your closet, throw away worn and obviously old pairs, even if they are your favorites. After all, Angelina Jolie wouldn't be seen in ballet flats with holes in the soles, would she? Of course not. From now on, those same rules apply to you. Visibly worn shoes have got to go—but if only the soles or heels are damaged, while the uppers are OK, there's a chance that a good shoe repairman or cobbler could make your old shoes look new.

Keep in mind, also, that "old" is relative. If you have a pair of shoes from two, three, five, even ten years ago that still are in great shape, that still have a style you like, and that still look good on your foot, keep those even if their exact design isn't "in." Fashion right now is so cyclical—something we'll talk about in the next chapter—that those shoes are sure to come back, and you'll look right on trend wearing them again.

Without jumping to the subject of the next chapter—how style changed from decade to decade—you can keep older shoes if their shape harks back to something iconic. A classic peep-toe pump is a great example. These shoes are all the rage now but were also popular in the seventies and early nineties. Platform pumps, flat pumps, forties-style T-strap heels, and ballet flats are all pretty much constantly in style and are safe to keep in your closet. If they go "out" it will probably be only for a brief moment—and when they come back in, you'll be armed and ready!

Of course, there's an exception to this rule too: high-fashion shoes. Designers sometimes go a bit wild when they design really conceptual shoes for runway and couture, like the Prada tailfin shoes released in January 2012. Since these shoes were never truly "in style," they'll never truly go out, either.

Building a solid shoe closet is relatively easy. You can never go wrong with shoes in nude, black, and metallic—especially in the styles described above, or with a round or pointy toe in a flat, stacked heel, low heel, or traditional high heel.

In terms of fabric, there is definitely a line between what you should wear during the day and what's worn at night. Though some, like patent and leather, work for both, day shoes are primarily of lighter, more textured material (like suede), while night shoes are usually more delicate material (such as satin or fabric) and tend to be more striking visually (such as a stiletto or a metallic). As usual in fashion, there are tons of acceptable variations—these are just guidelines! But when you're surveying your shoes, the same rules apply as with clothing: How do these shoes fit into your lifestyle? What's working for you? What are you missing?

# ...And Accessories!

ACCESSORIES PROVIDE A QUICK (and cheap!) way to create movie-star style, especially once you've crafted a go-to closet of clothes and shoes. There's lots of opportunity for starlet sparkle. For example, diamond drop earrings (Swarovski makes affordable crystal earrings in this style) are perfect for day or night, as are cuff bracelets and stackable bracelets. You can amp up the "volume" for night by adding more sparkle and bracelets, or both! Waist belts are a great accessory to make many an outfit stand out. Since classic movie-star glamour is about showing your curves in a classy way, having a few belts in colors that match your wardrobe and flatter your figure by defining your waist is excellent. I love that trend! Keep in mind that like shoes, accessories are relatively safe from going in and out of style. Though some styles are definitely cyclical—take the floppy hat, for example, which seems to show up more often than it disappears—most styles are fashionable for long periods of time. Some, like the hoop earring, are pretty much constantly in style, though some variations or details (like size) may change. Don't worry too much about whether your jewelry is silver or gold; it's acceptable to mix metals as long as it looks intentional. (Typically, mixing gold and silver bangles is fine, but wearing gold shoes with a silver bag rarely works.) Metals are another example of a cyclical trend—silver was in for the nineties, gold is back today—though most of us do have a preference, owning and wearing more of one than the other.

LAST BUT NOT LEAST, it's important to remember—through all of this—that movie stars create their own style from head to toe, including not only their clothes, hair, shoes, and accessories but also how the pieces are put together for a unique style. Only Angelina looks like Angelina, only Audrey looks like Audrey, and only you look like you. Though it's completely glam to enjoy well-designed clothes, cultivating movie-star style is about more than color theory, logos, and red soles. It's about great style. Which, as I'll show you in the next chapter, can be found at any price! ★

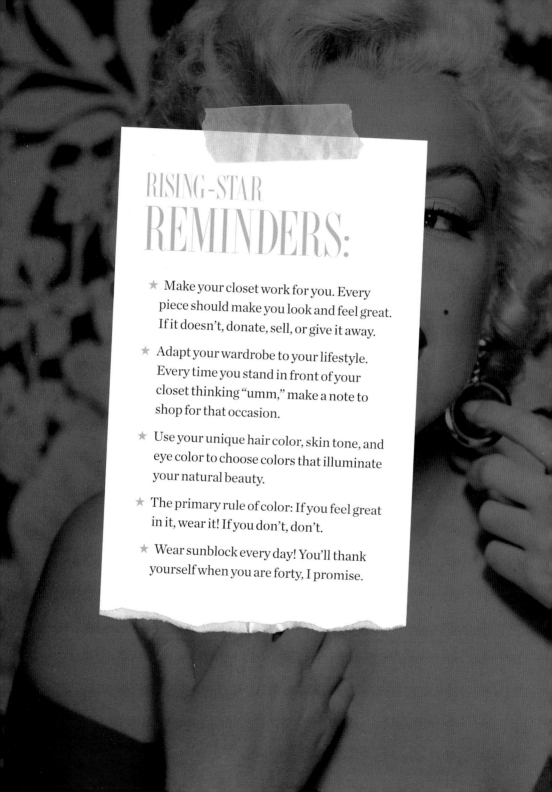

# RISING-STAR
# REMINDERS:

★ Make your closet work for you. Every piece should make you look and feel great. If it doesn't, donate, sell, or give it away.

★ Adapt your wardrobe to your lifestyle. Every time you stand in front of your closet thinking "umm," make a note to shop for that occasion.

★ Use your unique hair color, skin tone, and eye color to choose colors that illuminate your natural beauty.

★ The primary rule of color: If you feel great in it, wear it! If you don't, don't.

★ Wear sunblock every day! You'll thank yourself when you are forty, I promise.

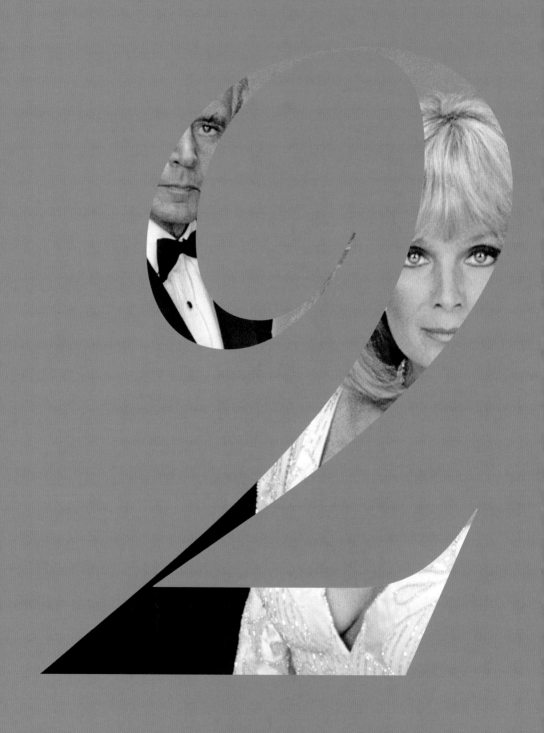

and know exactly where everything is. But if you love to look at your jewelry, it's OK to position the trays or organizers on a dresser or wardrobe in your bedroom as well.

## Shopping for Shoes

LET'S DISCUSS WHAT IS UNDOUBTEDLY EVERY LADY'S favorite sartorial subject—shoes! It used to be that a woman could get away with an inexpensive outfit as long as she had a nice bag and shoes. But nowadays the technology to make stylish shoes at a low price is better than ever, so options for "cheap" footwear are vast and offer really chic and wearable styles. Fast-fashion shoe resources like Aldo, Steve Madden, and Nine West offer up-to-the-minute fashionable shoes that won't break the bank. For an online option, try my favorite site, www.justfab.com. They forgo traditional brick-and-mortar stores, so they can keep retail prices down to $39.95! Look for cheap shoe options done in fabric, faux patent leather, and real suede, as they tend to look the most expensive. Fast-fashion chains are great for buying super-trendy shoes you plan to wear only occasionally. But for the everyday shoe you wear constantly, it's wise to invest in quality—so you won't end up buying new pairs every few months.

Finding a cheap evening-shoe option can be tricky, since evening shoes tend to be either an elegant satin or dazzling metallic. Try a shoe in a synthetic satin and faux metallic leather in a darker color that will blend into the background better and may not show any signs of faux material. But just like clothing, shoes made of synthetics may not allow your skin to breathe, so make sure to get the correct size or stick to something open and strappy, so there's room for your foot to breathe. Also, think about sleek and modern shapes; avoid a wide, square toe or anything too dowdy.

While I appreciate and adore the beauty of a Louboutin heel or the couture elements of a Roger Vivier pump, for most people they should remain in the über-luxury realm, unless you can get these shoes at 80 percent off. Saving your money and being able to take care of yourself in old age is more glamorous than

# HOW TO FIND A
# GREAT VINTAGE STORE

**I**f you are in a major city—like Los Angeles, New York, Chicago, Seattle, San Francisco, Washington, DC, Boston, Minneapolis—try searching online, including resources like Yelp. If the reviews are fairly good, hit it. If not, don't.

If you don't live in a major metro area, a technique I use is to find the artsy, "cool" area and ask around. An indie coffeehouse is a safe bet for vintage recommendations, as is a high-end department store like Saks or Bloomingdale's where the employees love clothes and will know where to shop in their town. Employees at general, big-box stores like Target might also be the ones to ask, but people at H&M and Zara will also be a good resource.

There is a difference between vintage and thrift. While thrift stores may have some great vintage pieces, strictly vintage stores usually have a more curated selection, which can result in faster finds. But if you're the kind of shopper who enjoys the hunt, a thrift store may be both fun and worth the time it takes to uncover a divine treasure.

## George's Favorite Vintage Stores

Vintage stores are a great source for cheap chic finds, special-occasion dresses, and formalwear that will look movie-star elegant forever. Here are my favorites!

### Decades, Inc.

This store is one of my absolute favorites because it is amazingly well curated and offers both vintage and current looks from top designers. The original Decades store has clothes from the 1950s through the 1990s, most of which are in great or mint condition.

Downstairs at Decadestwo there's a huge array of barely worn designer bags, jewelry, shoes, and clothes from the past few years, some of which is even current season. I have found so many fabulous finds in this place, for shoots, clients, and even myself!

# JEWELRY:
## *The Good, the Bad, and the Ugly*

### First the bad:

★ Rhinestones that look like plastic, not crystal or glass, are a sure sign of bad, fake jewels, particularly when they are glued onto a setting rather than set in prongs similar to real diamonds.

★ Your metal pieces should have some physical weight to them, since flimsy metal actually looks flimsy. For example, a great golden cuff needs to have some weight and substance to it, or you'll look like you're trying to get away with wearing the accessories from an old Wonder Woman costume.

★ Cheap finishes on jewelry will wear down quickly with use, so make sure from the start that you are not able to scrape off the finish on the jewels with your nail.

### Now the good:

★ When it comes to metal pieces that have an oxidized look to them or are even faux-aged, those generally tend to look like chic vintage jewelry (that you really only paid $6.99 for at H&M).

★ Enamel is an easy and cheap way to inject a shock of color into your look. Enameled accessories look great in vivid hues like turquoise and coral. Make sure that if any enamel pieces are glued in, the pieces are set in straight and securely and there's no excess glue bubbling up from the crevices.

★ For summer, accessories can be lighter weight and made from exotic-feeling materials like raffia and woven rope (these things generally come with a lighter price tag too!). Don't rule out certain pieces or colors because they have a more seasonal look. Cool tribal-style accessories woven with both natural and bright colors are generally a big trend on the runway during resort and spring collections and typically look fresh and bright when paired with a summery ensemble.

Ultimately, your entire ensemble will determine whether your jewels look chic or shocking, so stick with the "less is more" adage and keep your accessories to one statement piece, because when it comes to jewels, it's easy to have too much of a good thing.

## Inexpensive Jewels

WHEN IT COMES TO COSTUME JEWELRY, fast-fashion chains are amazing! The ironic but cool thing about fine jewelry is that even the small percentage of people who can afford real Cartier or Harry Winston oftentimes ends up wearing costume jewelry. Most stars wear it when traveling, because they don't want to risk losing their expensive items—or worse, having them stolen! With costume jewelry you never have that fear, aside from the sentimental value of a great piece. As far as getting dressed up or punctuating a casual look is concerned, costume jewelry gives you a ton of bang for your buck.

There is always a massive selection of things to comb through and find a gem or two. Layering three cheap necklaces together to make one big fabulous statement necklace almost always works. I was seated across from Helen Mirren at a dinner once and could not stop staring at her gorgeous diamond pendant. Of course, she is such an elegant woman I assumed it was real, but when I asked her about it, she said it was $9.99 from the mall! I fell in love with her at that moment. A simple "thank you" from Ms. Mirren would have been fine and very appropriately movie starrish, but she was honest and confident enough to share the origins of her cheap and fun little jewelry find, which in my eyes makes her even more fabulous. It really *is* all about the overall presentation and how you carry yourself.

Speaking of presentation, I often use black velvet stackable trays to display new, vintage, and costume jewelry at fittings and shoots. Most of the baubles I bring for a celebrity are a mix of fine jewelry and the latest offerings from fast-fashion chains, but it all looks simply gorgeous when presented on these plush trays. There are also black velvet jewelry organizers that can organize and display your jewelry. You can find the trays and the jewelry organizers at home/organization stores like Bed Bath & Beyond, HomeGoods, and The Container Store, for starters. You can also buy actual commercial displays at Acme Display online—that's where all the stylists get theirs! I think jewelry trays and organizers are great for your closet because you can label the outside

# *era-sistible* wardrobe

I OFTEN HEAR PEOPLE SAYING that they were "born in the wrong era," suggesting they would be so much happier if they were gussied up in a broad-shouldered 1940s frock or a sexy wiggle dress from the 1950s. I understand nostalgia and the romance of a bygone era, and I certainly appreciate the sartorial highlights from decades past, but the truth is that from the 1920s to the 1990s, fashion has essentially been on repeat, and as a result, women can dress according to any decade they want! How's that for great news? Even society's views on body types came full circle from the 1920s to the 1990s. Women in the 1920s wanted that prepubescent, board-straight body, and we saw the same desire for the string-bean frame during the heroin-chic phase that surfaced in the latter half of the 1990s.

And since everything has more or less been on repeat for the past decade or so, fashion is much less trend driven and more about dressing for your personal taste and body type. If a flare-leg jean looks fantastic on you, then why

# THE PAIN OF
# BEAUTY

Women have done pretty crazy things in the name of beauty. Though women don't wear hoop skirts or tight corsets very often anymore (except on Halloween), they do still torture themselves to look pretty. Wearing another woman's hair as extensions, injecting chemicals to minimize facial wrinkles, wearing six-inch stilettos that change the shape of your foot, and using laser techniques that keep your body from sweating are all just as unnatural as the "revolutionary" methods women used in the past, such as wearing arsenic and lead (both poison) as makeup.

Ultimately, movie-star style isn't about false beauty achieved by crazy methods or radical treatments. It's about looking amazing by highlighting your natural beauty. I urge you to think twice about any rash method of becoming "beautiful."

hide the flare legs until a fashion magazine says they're back "in"? A great-fitting pair of jeans, a Breton striped tee, and a pair of ballet flats are always in style and look even better when they flatter your best features.

For better or worse, when it comes to referencing a certain decade, there really are no rules anymore. Take aspects from the era you love and that suit your body type best—you can't go wrong when dressing by any of these decades, whether it's a direct reflection of vintage fashion or a mashup of a few different eras. Also consider the movie stars of the particular decade and how they managed to manipulate their shape with garments and technology introduced each year. The point is to have fun and flaunt your assets while also hiding your flaws.

In this chapter, I've taken each decade and pointed a spotlight at the clothes and the movie stars that shined brightest during the time. Delve into one decade or dabble in a few here and there (it's better not to make the look too literal, which seems like you're wearing a costume), but take snippets from the time that speaks loudest to you and helps you look your absolute best depending on your body type.

# 1920s: *The Boyish Babe*

**She's slim, straight, and devoid of any curves. Her chest is on the smaller side (B cup or smaller), and her arms and shoulders are delicate but toned.**

**BEST FEATURES:** Shoulders, décolletage, and arms; great calves and a beautiful poitrine (fancy French fashion speak for "chest").
**POSSIBLE PROBLEM AREAS:** Larger bottom, thicker middle, and upper thighs.
**MOVIE STARS WHO SHINED:** Clara Bow, Gloria Swanson, Lillian Gish, and Louise Brooks (page 64).

The silent-film era of the 1920s is when flappers sizzled on and off screen with their dramatic beauty and drop-waist frocks. But curves were not a part of the fashion equation in the twenties because women wanted a board-straight frame.

The 1920s' biggest stars, like Louise Brooks, Clara Bow, and Lillian Gish, created a linear silhouette by wearing drop-waist dresses, mid-calf-length skirts, and nonconstricting fabrics.

Though it wasn't apparent in their silhouette, some of these stars had curves and pear-shaped bodies—smaller on top, rounded shoulders, with fuller, rounded bottom halves.

If you have a pear shape, the twenties screen goddesses can be a great inspiration. A dress with a loose middle and a roomy or flowy lower half, hitting either mid-thigh or at shin length, is perfect for a pear shape because it hides middle, rear end, and upper thigh issues. Bare arms are a really big deal here, as showing them off is the best way to balance out the proportions of the look. If you're a B cup or smaller, a deep V neckline draws attention to the area and creates some necessary angles to balance out the roundness on bottom. Dare to go braless if you want; the women in the 1920s did. Many even went without any underwear—scandalous!

To make this look modern (because I am not suggesting you wear exactly

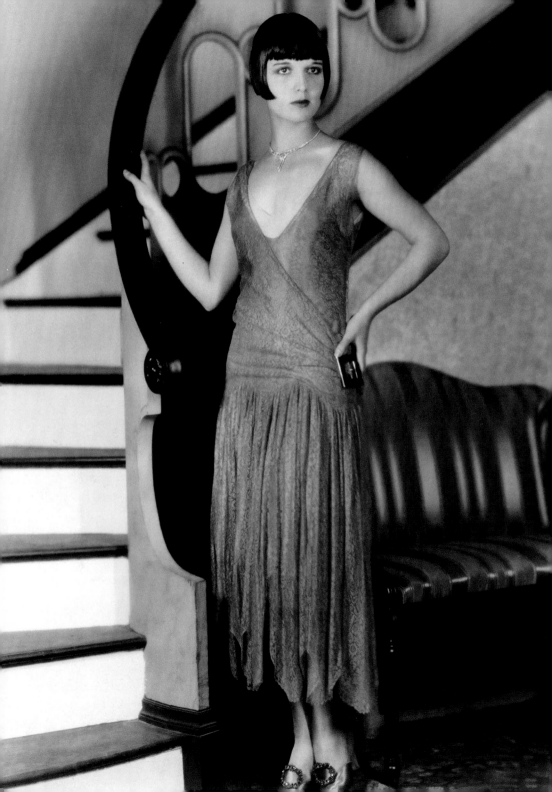

what the stars of the 1920s did, unless of course you are going to a costume party or have managed to find one of Ralph Lauren's gorgeous *Great Gatsby*–inspired dresses), try a longer tunic-style top paired with slim jeans or leggings.

And because a twenties-inspired silhouette is the most conservative of all movie-star looks, a high heel will go a long way. A heel (stiletto, if you can manage—remember, a platform sole always helps with comfort and balance) will take you from schlumpy to sexy in seconds.

# 1930s: *The Silver Screen Goddess*

**This woman is curvy and soft, with a full bust, small waist, elegant shoulders, and great calves. She is feminine but not quite an over-the-top bombshell.**

**BEST FEATURES:** Full bust, small waist, and developed shoulders.
**POTENTIAL PROBLEM AREAS:** Thicker legs and upper thighs, full hips, and full bottom.
**MOVIE STARS WHO SHINED:** Greta Garbo, Jean Harlow, Carole Lombard, Bette Davis, Marlene Dietrich (page 67), and Joan Crawford.

The 1930s ushered in an era when legendary movie stars began to appear on sets, making film and fashion history. Women like Greta Garbo, Jean Harlow, Bette Davis, and Joan Crawford were no demure silent stars; they had more of a brooding, dramatic, and sometimes even dark screen presence in their work and image.

This period is the pinnacle of Old Hollywood glamour, and was when the female form returned to fashion. Being slight and shapeless was not the look; this era celebrated the body with bias-cut gowns, cowl necklines, and sumptuous body-skimming fabrics like silk and satin punctuated with fur trims, rhinestones, and beading.

These screen stars had natural and curvy figures, and the fluid, slinky dresses they wore highlighted their gorgeous shape. The bias cut—fabric cut on the diagonal so that a garment moves with the wearer—was introduced to the world by fashion designer Madeleine Vionnet and became a popular cut in the 1930s. Bias-cut skirts and dresses are still ubiquitous today and work incredibly well on someone with an athletic build, because the fabric hugs the body and embraces the female form in a very natural way.

Jean Harlow was famous for wearing bias-cut dresses. She may seem like a hard act to follow, but the cut is really flattering on all body types and, more important, makes for a very comfortable fit. A bias-cut dress generally is just a flat panel of fabric across the tummy, so if you have any bulges in that area (and let's face it, who doesn't?) then don't forget your best friend—shapewear!

# 1940s: *The Pinup*

**Curves are back in full effect, and this woman fits the mold. She has narrow shoulders and killer legs and understands exactly how to flaunt them.**

**BEST FEATURES:** Slender legs, small bottom, and great calves.
**POTENTIAL PROBLEM AREA:** A body that's too straight up and down and is in need of some amazing curves!
**MOVIE STARS WHO SHINED:** Hedy Lamarr, Rita Hayworth, Jane Russell, Lana Turner, Lena Horne, and Betty Grable (aka "the girl with the million-dollar legs" and the "quintessential pinup," seen on page 68).

Skirt hems rose in the 1940s to save wool and money for World War Two, leaving legs exposed, creating a dramatic shift from the floor-length styles of the 1930s. Nylon hosiery was introduced to the masses, making perfect legs attainable by everyone.

The glamazons of the era such as Katharine Hepburn, Rita Hayworth, Lana Turner, and Ingrid Bergman (plus some very talented costume designers from the major studios) utilized the introduction of separates during this period to create very flattering silhouettes. The image these women projected was bold, severe, and at times even domineering. Clothing was used to create strong angles and extreme proportions to match their on- and off-screen personas.

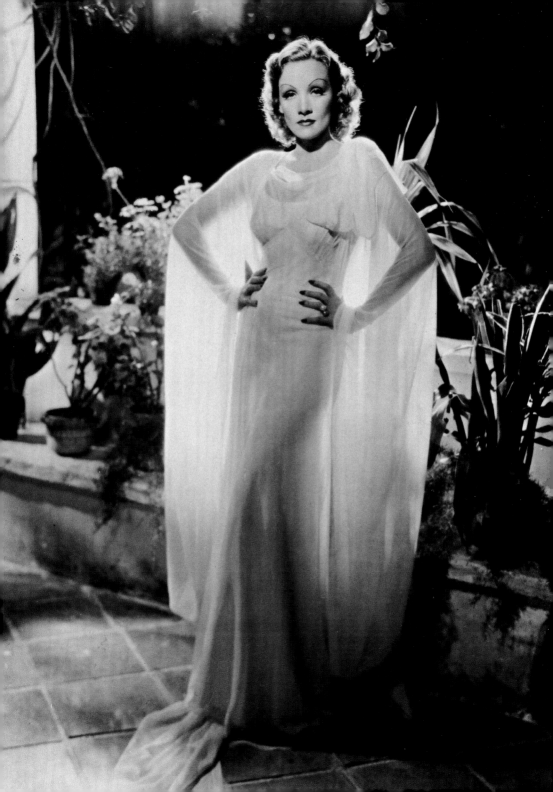

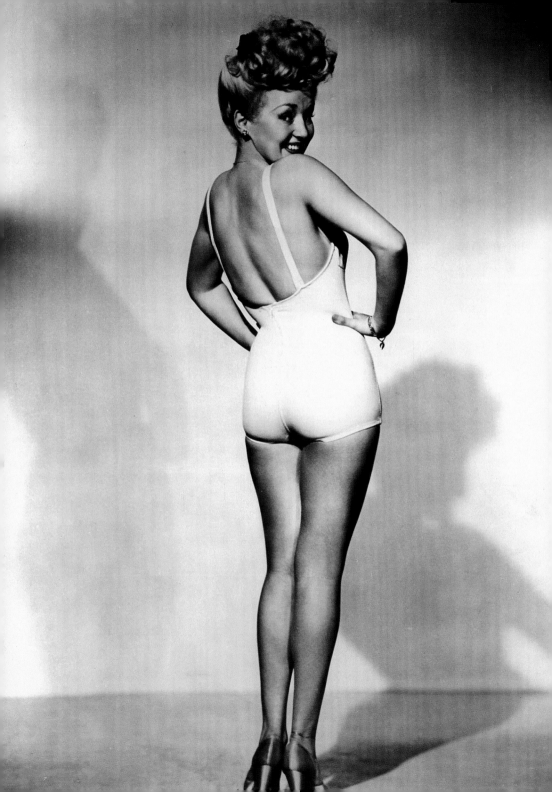

Details such as peplums on jackets were used to create a waist. Peplums make the hips look wider and the waist look smaller, drawing the eye in to create the illusion of a small, cinched-in waistline.

Whittle down a thicker waist, while also adding curves to an otherwise straight up-and-down figure, by taking a cue from the stars of the 1940s. Start integrating items into your wardrobe that add to the illusion of a slender waistline while accentuating your collarbones and shoulders and adding curves to the hip and chest area. An easy fix is a strong-shouldered blazer or jacket. A blazer draws attention to the outer shoulder area and keeps the eye up and out, while making the waist look smaller.

While skirt hemlines rose, that didn't mean women were walking around in minidresses. Skirts and dresses hit right around mid-shin, so if you have great calves but don't love your knee–to–upper thigh region, a 1940s-style skirt or dress may be perfect. Just use caution, because this length can come off as frumpy if you don't define a waist or show enough skin. Think light and with a little bit of movement.

# 1950s: *The Bombshell*

**In a word, voluptuous. She's got exaggerated curves on both the top and bottom and isn't afraid to show off her womanly figure.**

**BEST FEATURES:** Demure waist, large chest, and curves for day looks.
**POTENTIAL PROBLEM AREAS:** Broad shoulders, wide hips, and curves that need structured clothing to look defined and sexy.
**MOVIE STARS WHO SHINED:** Dorothy Dandridge, Elizabeth Taylor, Sophia Loren, Marilyn Monroe, Jane Russell (page 71), and Kim Novak.

The post-war era of the 1950s brought us movie stars with nipped waists and full bosoms, who fit the ideal of feminine and voluptuous. Any modern-day woman with a curvy figure can borrow some serious style tips from this group of bodacious beauties. Even the women who didn't quite have the kind of curves that were de rigueur in the day wore girdles and falsies to enhance their breasts. Strapless bras became popular, and in general, no one seemed to shy away from accentuating any trace of a robust chest and backside.

This era really had the most user-friendly fashion and still translates into how someone with a curvier figure can dress today. Primarily, it's about having structure in your clothing. Just as movie stars used girdles and bullet bras to accentuate their natural hourglass shape, women today use shapewear—essentially a return to corsets, just done in a more modern and less constricting way. When I worked with Salma Hayek on a photo shoot where corsets were involved (to make her look like a courtesan of Versailles), the actress instructed me to pull the apparatus tighter and tighter until it fit well, like a corset should. She understood that it's called "shapewear" for a reason and that, ultimately, sometimes beauty can be pain. Her determination to look exactly the part instantly sealed her as a movie star in my eyes.

When you choose a longer or fuller skirt, it is especially important to wear the proper proportions, so one doesn't walk away looking like a cream puff. The "sweater girls" of the time used second-skin, tight-fitting knitwear to really enhance their upper halves without showing any skin. This silhouette is easy to emulate today, whether you're busty or flat-chested. Have you heard of chicken cutlets? Not the kind you grill and eat but the jelly-like inserts that slip right into your bra cups and enhance the chest a bit more than any bra could on its own—and a far cry from the rolled-up socks the fifties girls would stuff into their bras for a similar effect. No matter what shape you are, don't shy away from body shapers, waist belts and cinchers, chicken cutlets, or even the occasional butt pad. Hey, I carry these things in my styling kit for clients all the time. In fact, my sister came over recently and started complaining about the size of her tummy. I brought her into my studio and had her put on a waist cincher that totally smoothed her belly. Her eyes were beaming with excitement about all the clothes she could wear again—all thanks to a simple piece of spandex!

Katy Perry is a great example of making classic 1950s styles look current—and has been, even way before she was a star. I met her back before she topped

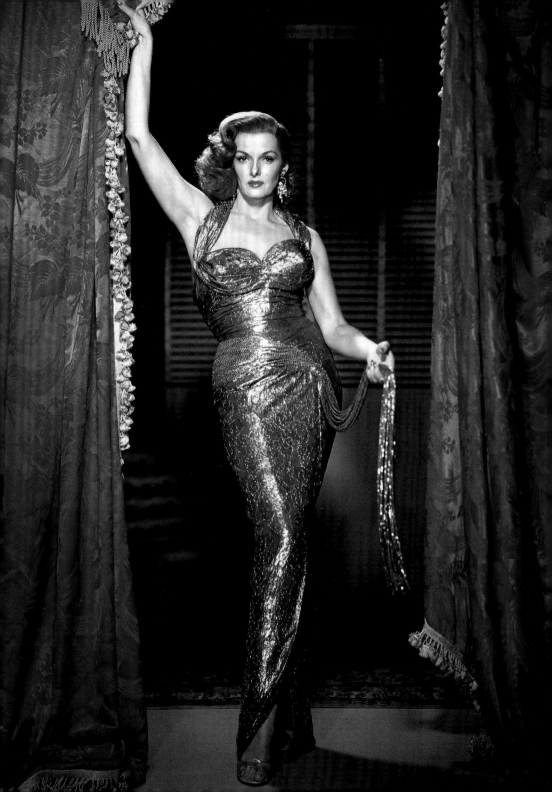

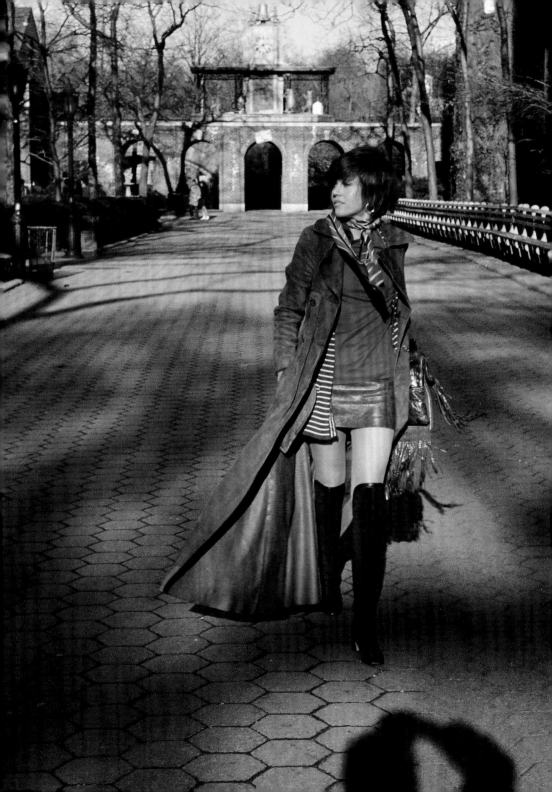

the charts (over and over again!). Even though she did not have access to the level of fashion designers she does today, she knew what looked best on her body. She requested a sweetheart neckline on her dresses and tops, knowing anything in that cut would be the most flattering on her bodacious bosom. Katy is also the perfect example of how anyone can look runway chic on a budget. She selected vintage pieces that made it look like she was wearing current (at the time) Lanvin! That she knew not only how to make herself look chic but that she could do it on a dime was one of the things I loved (and love) about her.

If you have a fuller bottom and want to embody 1950s style, try slipping on a pair of capri pants that hit a few inches above the ankle. The slender ankle area will provide a nice contrast and balance out curvy hips. Remember, we're not hiding anything, we're balancing and using a few easy decade-driven tricks to flatter, flatter, flatter! Creating a waist— with either the length of the clothes or a belt—helps hide a bigger bottom when wearing a full skirt, because it accentuates your body's natural curves and looks hot!

# 1960s: *The Leggy* (like Twiggy, but a bit more womanly)

**This swinging decade welcomed long, lean, and gorgeous gams. Skirts rose higher, and it was hard to notice anything but a lady's beautiful legs.**

**BEST FEATURES:** Legs, legs, legs! Also, nice, sleek, and slim arms.
**POTENTIAL PROBLEM AREAS:** A more rectangular body, thicker through the middle, possibly with a fuller chest.
**MOVIE STARS WHO SHINED:** Audrey Hepburn, Doris Day, Mia Farrow, Natalie Wood, Shirley MacLaine, Jane Fonda (at left), and Ann-Margret.

Love your legs? Then look to the actresses of the 1960s when dressing your inner movie star. This decade was all about the legs—think hot pants, miniskirts, shift dresses…

This was the first time that an underweight woman was considered the standard of beauty. (I mean, come on, Twiggy!) Consider also Audrey Hepburn's ultra-thin frame, which was slimmed down further when she pulled on a pair of black capri pants and a second-skin black turtleneck. Granted, these women were thin from top to toe, but the sixties silhouette works for someone who regards her arms and legs as her best assets and wants to downplay a rounder middle.

Someone with an apple-shaped body can benefit from the styles of the sixties and the carefree yet still-polished manner in which these movie stars wore them. If your waist and torso aren't your favorite body parts, an A-line dress that hits about mid-thigh will smooth out the middle area and really highlight your legs. The A-line shape will skim right over a thick middle and allow some breathing room whether you're working, dancing, or just going about your day in style—and most important, comfort.

When showcasing legs, heels will only help the cause, making the line of the leg even more long and sleek. Pair the dress or skirt with a wedge or heel to add height and length to the lower half of the body. Go for something with a vamp (aka the top of the foot) that's low and hits closer to the start of the toes—now is the time for a little toe cleavage! The lower cut will create the illusion of a much longer leg. Avoid a shoe with an ankle strap that cuts off the line of the leg. (The exception to this is if you have ultra-long legs. Essentially, if you're a short lady or have short legs, ankle straps are a don't; if you're tall, then these are a do.)

Remember, this decade is all about the legs, so choose a shoe that makes your leg look best. Darker pantyhose or opaque black tights will also make the leg look slimmer and longer. When I was styling Zooey Deschanel, there was an ever-present pair of black tights at all fittings. She loves a great sixties-style dress that shows off her legs and understands that adding opaque black tights makes her legs look even more lean. They've now become a signature part of her style!

I also remember working with Gwen Stefani on a photo shoot in the late 1990s. We were told that she preferred long pants or a full-length skirt because she knew even back then that showing off her legs was not exactly her best look. You see, even movie-star-status ladies manipulate their fashion to put their best face forward. Gwen started to show off her legs as she became more comfortable with them, but in the meantime she managed to develop mega-star style that many of us can admit to having followed. Today, she looks amazing not only because of her increased confidence but also because she worked very, very hard to get into top physical shape. (Even more inspiration!)

Gwen now embodies sixties style when she wears fishnets with high shorts or a mini. But fishnets aren't just for rock stars! When worn in colors like brown, dark tan, or nude, fishnets can make the leg look svelte and shapely. In fact, nude fishnets are a cool alternative to nude hosiery for women who want the bare-leg look without actually having bare legs. Wear black fishnets sparingly as they can look a little too severe and can easily slip into *Cabaret* territory.

Another way to highlight those gorgeous gams is with a pair of sleek, chic pants. Notice I said "chic." A pair of jeans with stretch (I will NOT call this a jegging) will give the illusion and effect of a legging or a yoga pant but will be more substantial and sophisticated. Think about a quirky mod silhouette, where the legging is cut off just above the ankle, a dainty ballet flat, and an adorable A-line or swing coat over a simple striped three-quarter-sleeve shirt. The look is classic *Breathless* (a great sixties French film—see it, if only for the splendid style) and works on almost any body type. If stripes aren't working for you, then any semifitted, round-neck shirt will do. Think about using a bold, solid color for that appropriately 1960s color-blocking effect.

I want to reiterate that this look should be worn with a sleek pair of pants or jeans, NOT leggings, yoga pants, or God forbid, the j-word.

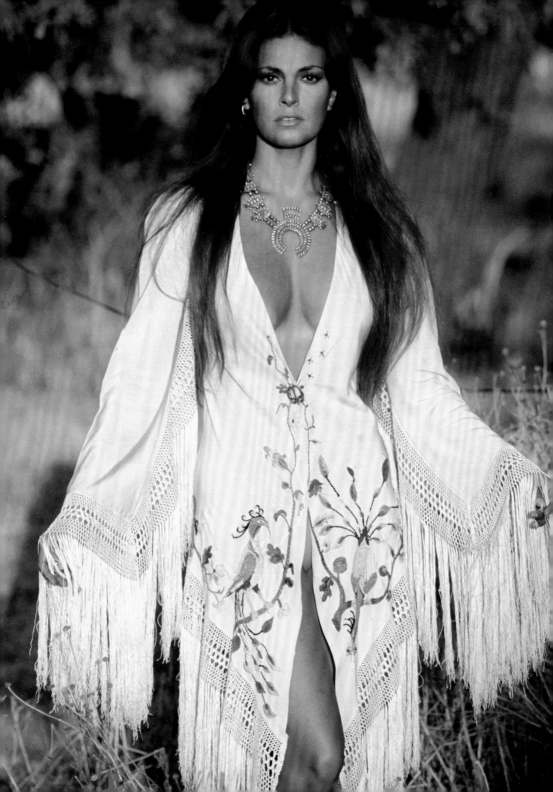

# 1970s: *The Natural* (no undergarments required)

**Enter the era of the all-natural, tanned, and trim golden girl. She's got a toned frame, long limbs, easygoing personality, and an effervescent smile.**

**BEST FEATURES:** Pretty much everything—what a lucky girl!

**POTENTIAL PROBLEM AREA:** OK, no body is perfect (thank goodness). If there is an area this girl should watch, it's having too much of a good thing and a little too much jiggle. The era was all about au naturel, which is great in theory but can be a little too free and loose for modern day.

**MOVIE STARS WHO SHINED:** Jacqueline Bisset, Candice Bergen, Raquel Welch (at left), Barbra Streisand, Goldie Hawn, Katharine Ross, Ali MacGraw, Diane Keaton, and Diana Ross.

Natural, lean, and athletic was the body type that most of the movie stars of the 1970s put forth. They could pretty much wear anything, and did! But though the women were thin and toned, there was an unaffected look to their bodies, nothing like the overdone yoga arms and emaciated frames (not to mention surgical *enhancements,* cough, cough) that are considered desirable today.

But the decade wasn't just about denim. Loose and flowy pieces that emulate fifties style work perfectly on a thin frame, just as they do for anyone who needs to hide a slight figure flaw. Talk about playing with proportions: pair skinny jeans with a breezy, blousy peasant-style top. The top is roomy, while the silhouette stays sleek on the bottom. A boho or peasant-style top also hides midriff and tummy issues and creates the illusion of a thinner upper thigh.

Maxi-length skirts and dresses are also forgiving and can look quite elegant. The long and flowy shape creates a vertical line from hip to heel. Pair it with something fitted to keep proportions balanced. If your top ends lower than your waist, try tucking it in or tying it up in an easy knot, to define the waist. A sleek wedge or platform instantly dresses up this look and is certainly more chic than a flimsy flip-flop.

Forgiving fabrics like ruched jersey and the wrap dress that Diane von Furstenberg made famous also became increasingly popular during the 1970s. Von Furstenberg's wrap is still a spectacular option for women of every body type today.

The decade also saw a lot of oversized accessories—think wide-brimmed floppy hats, sunglass frames the size of movie screens, and boho-style bags with colorful adornments or details. These pieces will work well to minimize any large feature. A round face can look smaller with the right pair of oversized sunglasses, and a wide-brimmed hat balances out broad shoulders and hips. Larger accessories in general will make anything next to them appear smaller in relation. Just don't use more than one at once, or you'll look like you raided Carly Simon's closet!

# 1980s: *The Super Woman*

**This lady can have it all—the career, the marriage, and the kids. She is toned, athletic, and strong. She took advantage of the fitness boom, and it shows.**

**BEST FEATURES:** Athletic build, broad shoulders, great arms, and for the first time, a focus on fantastic abs!

**POTENTIAL PROBLEM AREA:** Overly muscled arms and legs may not always look feminine or glamorous.

**MOVIE STARS WHO SHINED:** Michelle Pfeiffer, Kim Basinger, Sigourney Weaver, Kathleen Turner, Susan Sarandon, Jamie Lee Curtis (at right), Melanie Griffith, Diane Lane, Meryl Streep, and Jessica Lange.

Welcome to the decade of the power suit and spandex! Women had power all over the place, from their boxy jackets to the size of their shoulder pads, and though we wince at some of the era's styles, there are some great takeaways that can help dress someone with an athletic build or buff bod. The 1980s also welcomed the idea of self-expression through fashion. Think about how much variety there was—everything was good to go, from oversized separates to

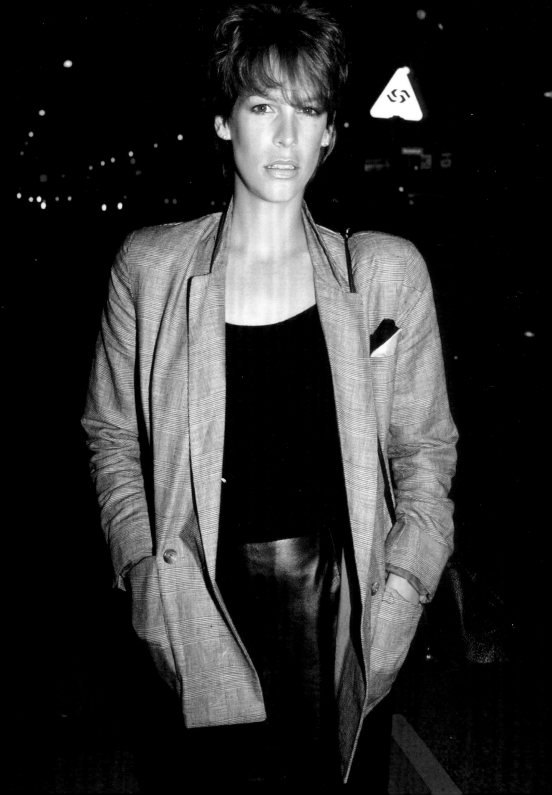

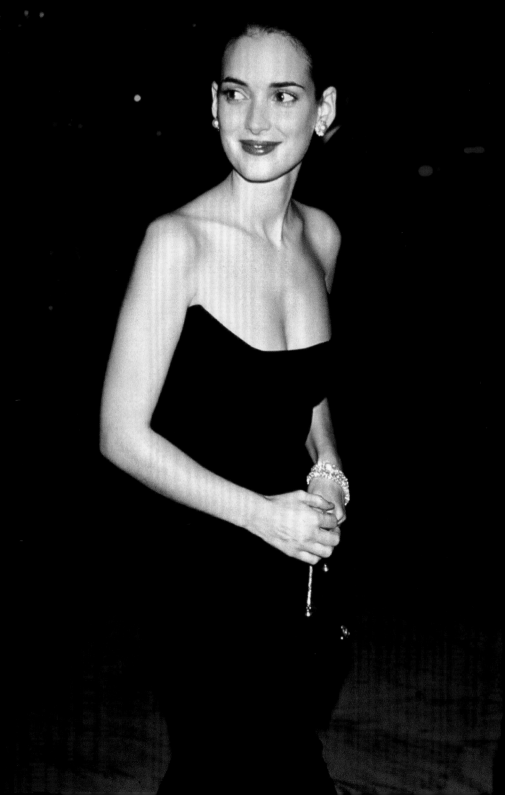

New Wave, preppy, goth, metal, and the *Miami Vice* looks! There was so much going on, it takes more than a minute to wade through all of it to find the style hallmarks that are still inspiring today.

A great icon of the eighties that still works today is the classic motorcycle jacket, immortalized then by Madonna, who loved to pair hers with leggings and short poufy skirts. Take a cue from the way Madonna did it and wear the leather jacket with something soft and romantic, such as over a maxidress or with a cute, short skirt.

There are so many adorable takes on the motorcycle jacket these days that it's hard not to find something that suits you. You can eschew traditional leather and go for denim; or do it up in a print, like a fun floral pattern; or pick something where the front has a cool, colorful knit and the sleeves are sleek and black. Designers constantly have interpretations of the motorcycle jacket in their collections, and most remain fashionable after their trendy time has passed. But the classic motorcycle jacket will always be in style.

# 1990s: *The Simple Girl* (with a great bod)

**This lady is built a bit like a lollipop, meaning the body type is all about the breasts. Her full and perky chest is further accentuated by a thin frame.**

**BEST FEATURES:** The full chest and long, lean legs.

**POTENTIAL PROBLEM AREA:** The body type can look a little top-heavy. Big chests may be desirable to many people, but it's important to keep it balanced so you walk out of the house looking tasteful, not trashy.

**MOVIE STARS WHO SHINED:** Nicole Kidman, Julia Roberts, Halle Berry, Annette Bening, Sharon Stone, Meg Ryan, Sandra Bullock, Drew Barrymore, Demi Moore, Winona Ryder (at left), Uma Thurman, and Angela Bassett.

The look of the 1990s was a total backlash to the materialism of the 1980s, brought on by a decade of sleek and controlled minimalism. Clothing took a turn toward understated, drapey, oversized, comfortable, and ultimately simple, which felt like "anti-fashion" fashion.

The minimalist aesthetic works well on someone who's a bit top-heavy, because there's nothing to draw attention to that part of the body. Stick with understated yet body-conscious clothes that skim the body but don't squeeze you too tightly. Soft, neutral colors like light gray, charcoal, nude, and ivory further temper a large chest and help balance the entire look.

Look at the movie stars of the day like Halle Berry, or even the Amazonian supermodels like Cindy Crawford and Naomi Campbell (OK, maybe they aren't exactly Amazonian, but compared to the reed-thin models who walk today's runways, they seem like voluptuous Venus de Milos). They all have ample chests and donned minimal pieces in neutral or solid colors to keep things tasteful (most of the time). Julia Roberts is a perfect example of good 1990s style. She wore (and still wears) tons of Armani, opting for understated, easy pieces that let her movie-star appeal shine through.

When it comes to necklines, you can wear something slightly fitted, body-conscious, and minimal without looking tacky. Take a cue from the clean and modern Calvin Klein aesthetic, which also hit its stride during this decade. Go for bold, solid colors, necklines that skim just under the collarbone, and sleeveless styles that show off your great arms.

For pants or a skirt, the sky is the limit. But remember, you're working to temper the top of your body, so wearing something tight and skinny down below will only make your top look bigger. Play with the pieces to strike the right balance between big breasts and being all-out bodacious. ★

# ERA MASHUP

While dressing by decade can be a streamlined approach to injecting some surefire style into your wardrobe while also appropriately suiting your body type, mixing and matching elements from each decade is fun and two, sometimes three times as fabulous! ★ Because the majority of original ideas in fashion occurred between the 1920s and 1990s, we've sort of been living in a mashup of all of those eras ever since, taking elements from each time period and making them work in new, interesting, and more-modern ways. It's not about trends these days as much as it is making the pieces that suit your body and personality work for you, and sometimes that means mixing it up! ★ Don't be afraid to combine, match, and mash up your decades to create an original idea with an individual style spin. So many specific items from different decades run parallel to one another, and variations pop up years later. It's a fun little history lesson to see how clothing evolves (or doesn't) and how fashion is indeed very cyclical. If you fancy yourself a twenties girl for the aesthetic and way the silhouettes suit your frame, you may very well also be a sixties girl in certain ways. Here are various ways to mash up decades and style items accordingly to fit your figure and personal style.

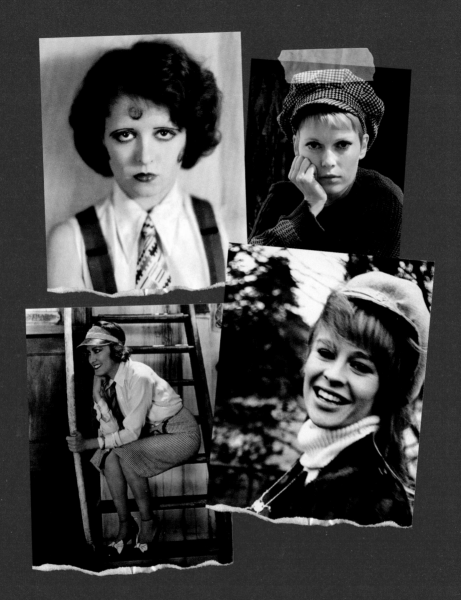

**1920s tomboy meets 1960s mod:** Both decades reflected many of the same boyish elements seen in drop-waist dresses, loose shift dresses, round-toe Mary Jane–style shoes, and hostess pants, as well as the no-fuss little black dress debuted by Coco Chanel in the twenties.

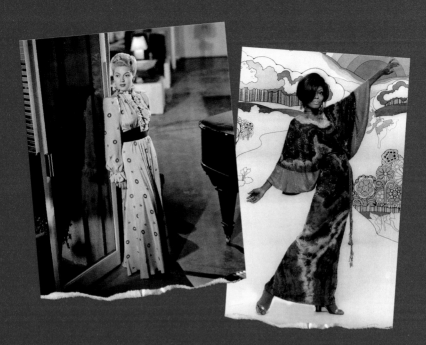

**1940s pinup meets 1970s boho babe:** The decades may seem different, but think about platform shoes with T-straps and ankle straps that debuted in the 1940s and appeared again in a big (and glittery!) way on the disco floors of the 1970s.

**1950s bombshell meets 1980s prepster and party girl:**
The 1980s were a mashup of various styles all their own, but a few key items really stick out. Many of them were borrowed from the very polished look of the 1950s, but this time thrown together in a punky and eclectic kind of way.

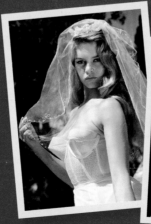

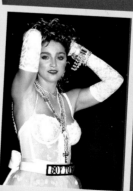

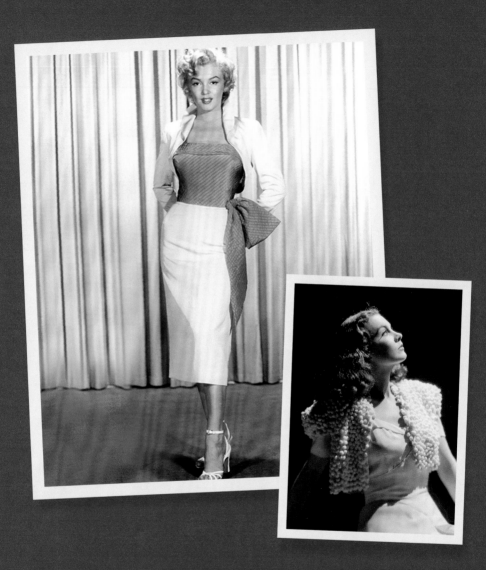

**Who can forget the cropped bolero-style jacket?**
The style first became popular during the 1930s, returned in the
1950s and 1960s, and then came back yet again in the 1980s.

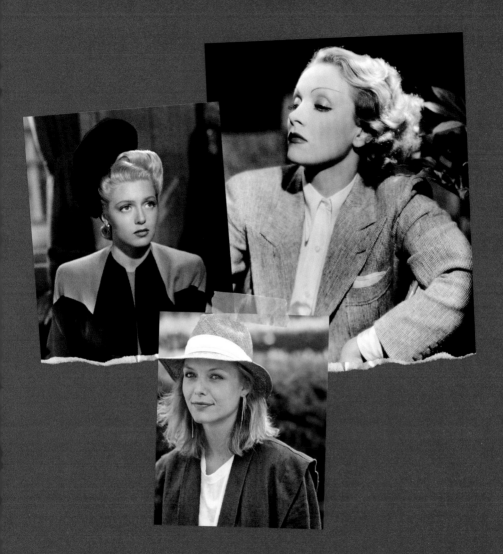

**Strong shoulders** (think exaggerated shoulder pads) and power dressing were big in the 1980s. The style was a nod to the strong shoulders from the 1940s as well as the 1920s and 1960s, when a small group of women donned the menswear look.

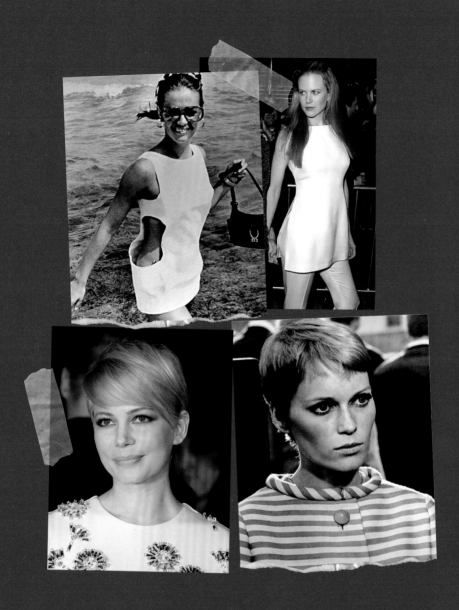

**The mod look** comes back into fashion all of the time. Tom Ford referenced it in the 1990s, and Marc Jacobs uses the look frequently, both in his namesake collection and in his designs for Louis Vuitton.

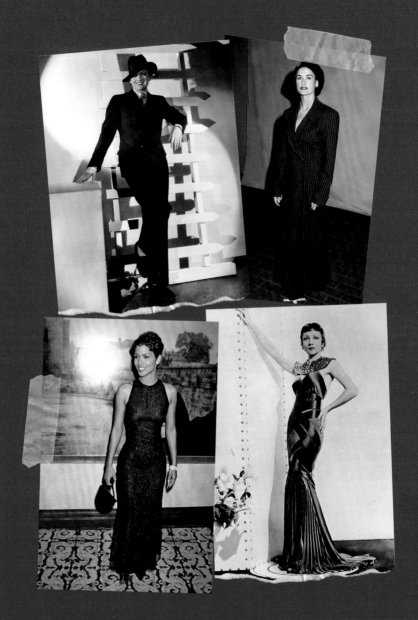

**1930s screen diva meets 1990s minimalist:** Think pinstripe
trousers and sharp, strong cuts on dresses from the 1930s, and
mash that up with the similarly bold line and angles of 1990s suits
(hello, Mr. Armani) and body-conscious dresses.

The heavily textured and patterned **baby-doll dresses** and lush velvets and brocades from the 1960s came back in a grungy-yet-sweet way when Anna Sui brought the look back during the 1990s.

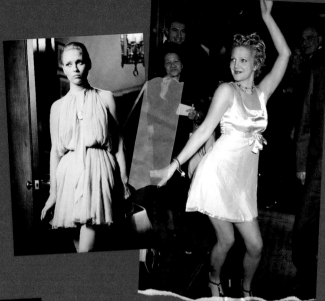

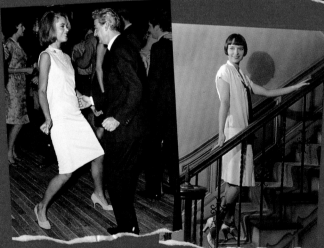

**The 1960s** revisited many past decades as well as set the pace sartorially for future styles to come. Besides the **boyish cuts borrowed from the 1920s**, which created a shapeless silhouette around the female form, we also saw wide-leg, low-slung pants similar to the femme fatales of the 1930s and 1940s.

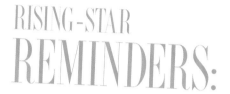

# RISING-STAR
# REMINDERS:

★ Don't worry about trends. You can always incorporate parts of trends in shoes and accessories, but you should really focus on what styles look best on your body.

★ Fashion is fluid! Feel free to mix and match looks from the past that best suit your body type.

★ Dressing head to toe in styles from one particular era can look like a costume. Combine vintage or throwback pieces with more-modern elements to make the classic look contemporary.

★ Movie-star style is timeless. Take cues from the leading ladies of the twentieth century to make your look unique, yet iconic.

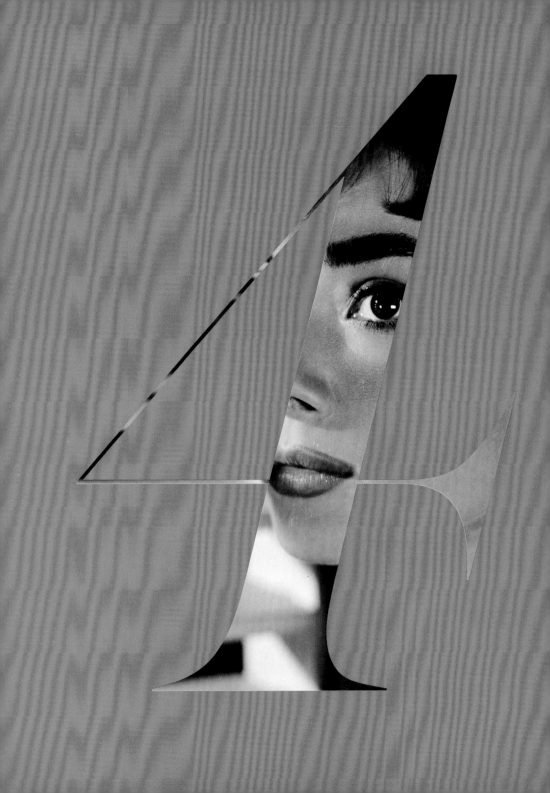

# era-sistible
# *beauty*

N FILM AND TELEVISION SETS, as well as fashion shoots, actresses and models get called to "hair and makeup" instead of just to "hair" or to "makeup." At most fashion shoots and television sets that I've worked on, the whole team of hair, makeup, and styling is called "the Glam Squad." The first time I ever heard that, I laughed out loud because the guy who said it—and this is typical—was a buff, manly assistant director. Today, it makes me feel sort of like a superhero: Never fear, the Glam Squad is here!

Whether it's an A-lister on a film or a model just starting out on a shoot, all women in the business of looking elegant, beautiful, and movie-star chic have their hair, makeup, and styling done almost simultaneously, by a team of people working together toward a single goal. Because we're trying to get you red-carpet ready, you should approach your beauty look—what we stylists call hair and makeup combined—the same way. Whether you're walking the red carpet or down the street, an effortlessly beautiful look requires hair and makeup that match. If your hair is crazy or your makeup is overdone, you'll look like a hot mess—guaranteed.

It should come as no surprise that I think the most gorgeous beauty looks are inspired by the leading ladies of the past. It's very simple to recycle vintage trends in hair and makeup with slight updates to create an overall effect that's chic and original today. As with fashion, the rules on makeup and hair have disintegrated into such an anything-goes world that nothing ever truly goes "in" or "out."

In addition to covering the beauty looks of the past that were glamorous then and can be glamorous today, I'll show you how to mix, match, and update particular trends so you can experiment with classic looks that stand out in a crowd yet look chic and completely on trend.

This might be stating the obvious, but your haircut and how you style it can often be the dividing factor between appearing elegant and put together versus messy and all over the place. A great haircut will not only suit your face shape and features but, just as important, work for your hair texture (which changes based on environmental and genetic factors) and reflect your personality. Because there are *so* many variables in hair, I'm not going to tell you what to do with the cut itself. However, I will give you advice on how to adapt classic looks from the past so you make the most out of that great cut you have.

When trying out classic styles, keep in mind that, like your weight, hair fluctuates. It can change texture, flexibility, hold, and length constantly based on what's going on environmentally, so if a style you try doesn't quite work today, it might tomorrow. Don't hold back. If you see something that you think is fun, cute, or even daring, try it!

Sleep in pin curls or rollers (today, there are soft ones available, so don't use the old hard ones your mom probably has!) to see if your hair will have rolling waves in the morning—or come out so limp that you think you dreamed the whole thing. Try a purple shadow or a dark lipstick at the makeup counter that you've never tried before. It might make you look like death—or it could totally

# HOW TO GET A
# GREAT HAIRCUT

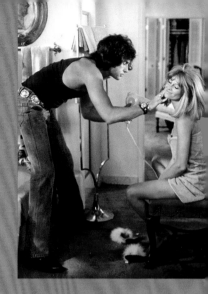

Here's a hard truth: If you have a haircut that's not working for you, it's either your fault or the hairstylist's fault. Period. Either you didn't tell the hairstylist information he or she needed (say, that your hair gets frizzy the minute there's any whiff of humidity), you insisted on a cut that won't work for your hair texture and the hairstylist gave in, or the hairstylist is just bad.

A lot of women feel obligated to go to the hairstylist they have seen in the past, but they shouldn't. If you're going to a hairstylist who cuts your hair badly, you're essentially paying someone to make you look terrible for weeks or months at a time. That makes zero sense. If you're sitting reading this book with a bad haircut, you have two options:

1. Go to a new hairstylist, at a new salon. Get recommendations from friends whose hair always looks great or—better yet—a friend who has hair texture similar to yours.

2. Return to your hairstylist and tell him or her everything you know about your hair. Talk about the terrible perm you got in the sixth grade, or the reason you've been hesitant to cut your hair above your shoulders, or why you want to look like Reese Witherspoon. Don't worry about rambling on; sometimes there will be a nugget of information that the hairstylist can use to transform your hair completely. After all, they are paid to listen to you and make you beautiful—so get what you pay for!

# POLITICAL HAIR

From announcing women's liberation in the 1920s with short haircuts to the free-love long hair of the 1960s and 1970s, using your hair as a political message was common in the twentieth century.

Even today, I've heard girlfriends complain that men don't like women with short hair. I say, do what makes you feel glamorous! Men have no idea how much work maintaining, styling, and sporting a woman's hair involves every day. Regardless, your hair is none of his business. But that being said, most men do prefer long hair. I'm just saying!

surprise you by making your eyes pop or giving you sultry, siren lips.

Remember: A bad hairstyle can be brushed out or washed down the drain; horrid makeup can be taken off with a gentle cleanser and a good washcloth. But movie-star style does not happen by accident. Your hair and makeup may be trial and error now, but soon—with the help of history—your glamorous look will be tried and true.

# 1920s: *Feminine Rebels*

EVEN THOUGH WOMEN OF THE 1920s were trying to gain equality, most still wanted a feminine look. Finger waves are a sophisticated and sexy way to style a short bob. If you want a 1920s look for a special occasion, finger waves are perfect—but this style tends to look way too "done" for everyday wear.

Even today, wearing a bob can be tough. This cut tends to look great on younger women and can look sophisticated on older women, but women in between (say, thirty-five to forty) typically end up looking like they are trying to dress young, resemble a soccer mom, or (eek!) both. However, this cut can work wonders for women with naturally wavy hair and thin hair, so you shouldn't necessarily avoid it. But if you decide to sport a short, 1920s blunt bob, it's important to amp up sophistication by wearing more makeup, adding a side part, wearing it with bangs, or all of the above.

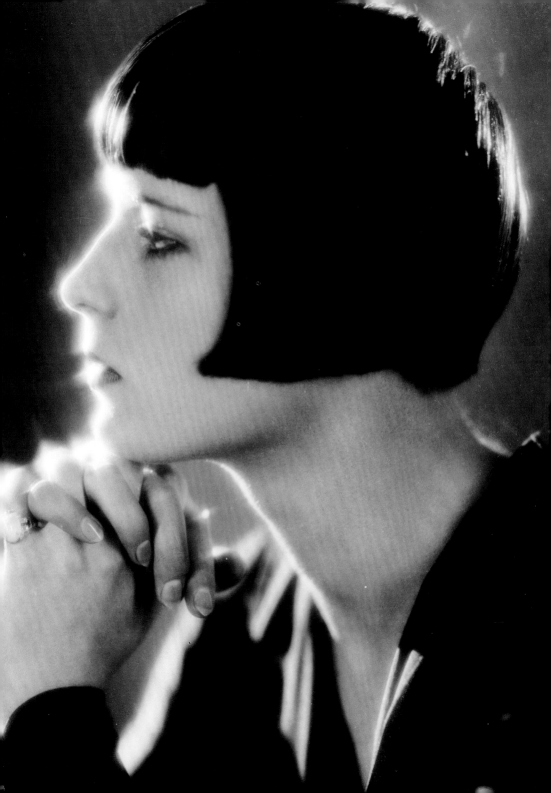

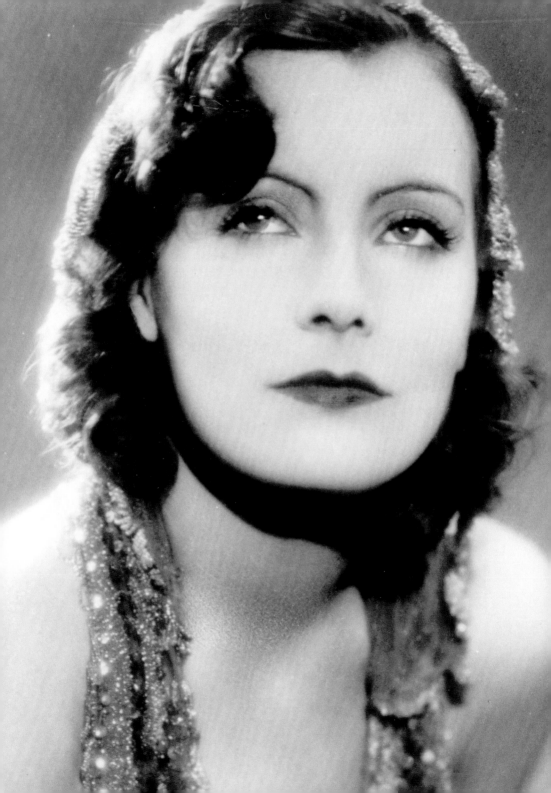

The overall style of the 1920s was boyish, and to balance that, makeup tended to be heavy. Most of us don't realize that women with short hair can wear more makeup than those with long hair (women with long locks and tons of makeup can look tarty).

If you're going for a classic silver-screen appearance, Clara Bow is great to mimic. Notice the sculpted, thin eyebrows, minimal eye makeup, and Cupid's bow lips, which were the main focus of this era, complete with dark red lipstick. This look is great when you want to make a striking, classic impression.

# 1930s: *The Tea Roses*

PEOPLE—EVEN STYLISTS—tend to lump the 1920s and 1930s together because the differences between these two decades are really very subtle. Whereas the twenties were all about a boyish look with heavy makeup, the next decade brought back softer feminine styles for clothes and hair, accompanied by more-natural makeup. Typically, women of this era grew out the short bob of the 1920s into a softer, longer cut that usually ended at chin length.

A big transition happened when the Great Depression hit. Since women could no longer afford to get their hair done, styles had to be done at home. Soft roller curls, perms, and natural waves became more popular, since these styles didn't require as much maintenance .

Makeup in the 1930s was also much more dramatic. A "tea rose" complexion—created by using foundation of the same name, ivory with a touch of pink—replaced the heavy-handed pallor of the 1920s. Women still used mascara heavily and sculpted their eyebrows thinly—just look at Greta Garbo—but they used much more eye shadow, applying vibrant colors like violet and green from the lid to the brow line. Women in the thirties also used Vaseline to make their eyebrows and eye makeup look shiny for day looks. In the thirties it was extreme; today it's common in photo shoots—and sometimes can work at night. In the daytime, however, it's absurd.

While a thirties makeup look could be great for a special occasion (especially one with a vintage theme), I would be wary of wearing it elsewhere because it is so dramatic. In contrast, the softer, wavier bob popular in this era works for many women with thin yet wavy hair and tends not to look soccer-mom-ish if styled correctly.

# 1940s: *Those Luscious Locks*

WHEN WOMEN WEAR VINTAGE HAIRSTYLES TODAY, most are trying to emulate the iconic looks of the 1940s. This era is my personal favorite, and I love styling models and celebrities in forties-inspired looks. This period is reproduced on the red carpet frequently because these styles are flattering and beautiful on nearly every woman. (And relatively easy to do!)

Beauty in this decade was about more than merely looking good. It was patriotic. In hair, women wore side parts because it complemented the styles of the day and created a flattering, feminine look. (I will always vote for a side part: It's sexier and more forgiving to your face!)

Women never looked frumpy in this era, which is one of the reasons I adore it. It simply wasn't acceptable to go out in public looking a mess, as it is today. Back then, the public tried to emulate stars' fashion and behavior, whereas now we turn to reality and tabloid shows to watch people fall from grace. You can only watch trashy behavior so long before you start to think it's OK—and it is *so not OK*. We're aiming higher than *Real Housewives* or the *Bad Girls Club*. If ladies in the forties had time to look good to wait in line for rations, you have time to look great at Starbucks. Period.

The most recognizable hairstyle of this decade is rolled curls, pinned to the sides, to the top of the head, or both. This can look costumey if you replicate it without either brushing out the curls or forgoing the top curl. Pinning back forties curls to the side can be a great day-to-night look, especially for women whose hair holds curl well. Emulating Veronica Lake's iconic curls,

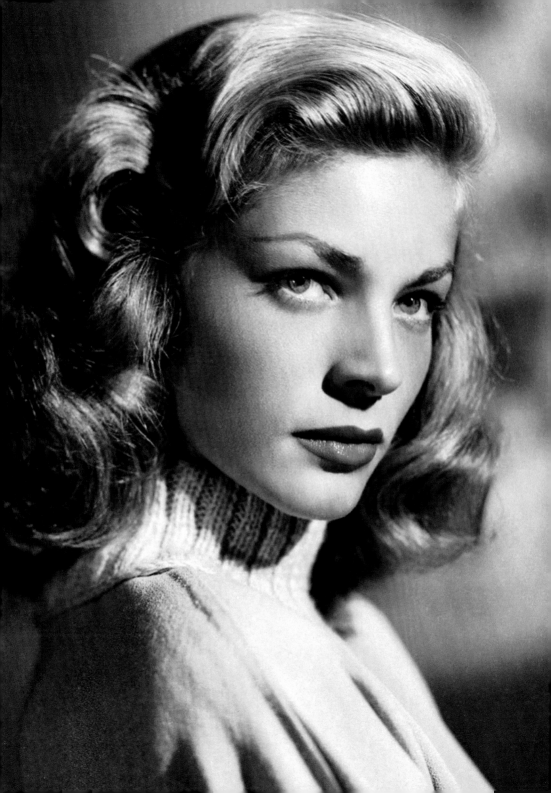

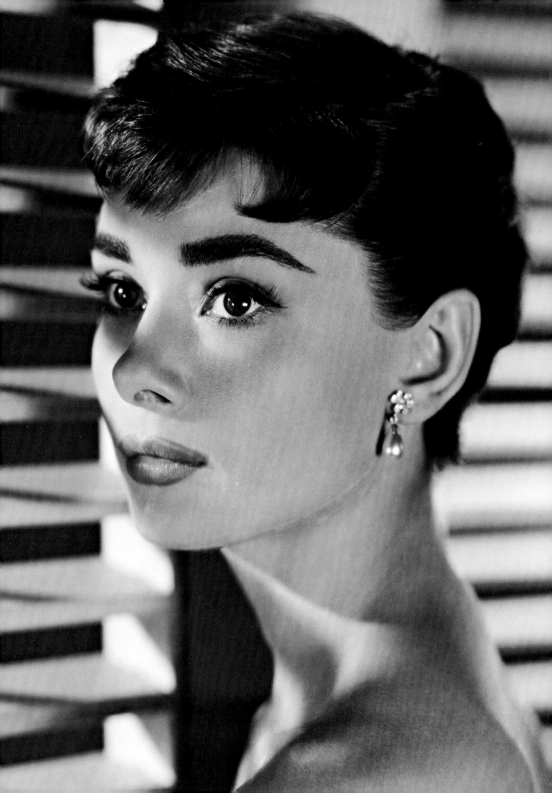

Lauren Bacall's long, loosely curled bob, or Betty Grable's soft waves is very common on the red carpet because these hairstyles hold their shape throughout a long event.

Like hairstyles of this era, makeup in the 1940s was more natural but not effortless. Women tended to pluck their brows into a high, pronounced arch and wear champagne-colored eye shadow to emphasize their eye color. Though lips were still red, the shades were much lighter than in past decades. The overall look was womanly, feminine, and sophisticated while still appropriate for dual roles at work and at home. Though forties-inspired hair and makeup each work on their own, don't wear both because that can make you look like you've watched too many Turner Classic Movies.

# 1950s: *Unnaturally Natural*

WOMEN AT THE START OF THE FIFTIES basically wore an adaptation of forties style, except with their roller curls brushed out, pinned to the sides and back rather than forward and front.

But in the middle of the decade, fashion and lifestyle magazines began printing spreads featuring glamorous women like Elizabeth Taylor and Audrey Hepburn, who—thanks to the new invention of hair spray making it possible—wore their hair in short, bouffant cuts and styles (of differing length, with Audrey's being shorter than Liz's). Since products that changed hair texture were suddenly widely available, this hairstyle was accessible to the average Jane.

The phrase "putting on a face" began in the 1950s because foundation and powder became widely available and affordable. The idea of "peaches and cream" was very popular, with pink hues, pastel shadows, lots of mascara, dark eyeliner, a wide arc in the eyebrow—and a crystal-clear complexion (if you didn't have it, you could fake it!) with an emphasis on looking natural.

I personally think 1950s makeup is the most transformative and accessible for women today. Wearing a neutral (think champagne-colored) eye shadow with thick black eyeliner and lots of mascara will make anyone's eyes pop, especially if you create a peachy foundation to offset it. (If you have a clear complexion, you are a lucky girl and can skip the foundation, though you might need a touch of blush, concealer, or even bronzer to get a warm glow.)

The fifties look emphasizes the eye beautifully without screaming, "Oh my God, I have so much makeup on!" The 1950s did a great job of looking natural without actually being natural, a look I am a huge fan of, both on the red carpet and in everyday life.

## SABRINA

If you want to see classic 1950s style, watch the 1954 version of *Sabrina* with Audrey Hepburn and Humphrey Bogart. I won't spoil the movie's plot for you (though there's a reason it was remade in the 1990s, ahem), but note how Audrey's hair changes throughout the movie. It not only matches what happened in the 1950s but applies to today as well.

When Audrey's character Sabrina is a girl, she wears her hair up, in a ponytail, with blunt bangs. But once Sabrina returns, as a woman … well, let's just say her hair isn't exactly girly any longer!

In the 1950s, Audrey Hepburn changing her hair in the movie (and in real life) was symbolic because it was acceptable to have long hair only if you were a young girl. At that time, once you were old enough to be considered a woman, you cut your hair into a shorter, more sophisticated style. I think this remains true today, even though some women seem to think you can have long hair forever!

# 1960s: *The Big Bang*

THIS DECADE WAS ALL ABOUT VOLUME, VOLUME, VOLUME—even though the styles radically changed from beginning to end. It's easy to see the transition on one of my favorite vintage television shows, *That Girl*. There was truly a drastic switch: At the beginning of the show in 1966, Thomas wore a big bouffant with a flip at the ends, and by the end—just five years later, 1970—she was sporting long, loose, sexy hair.

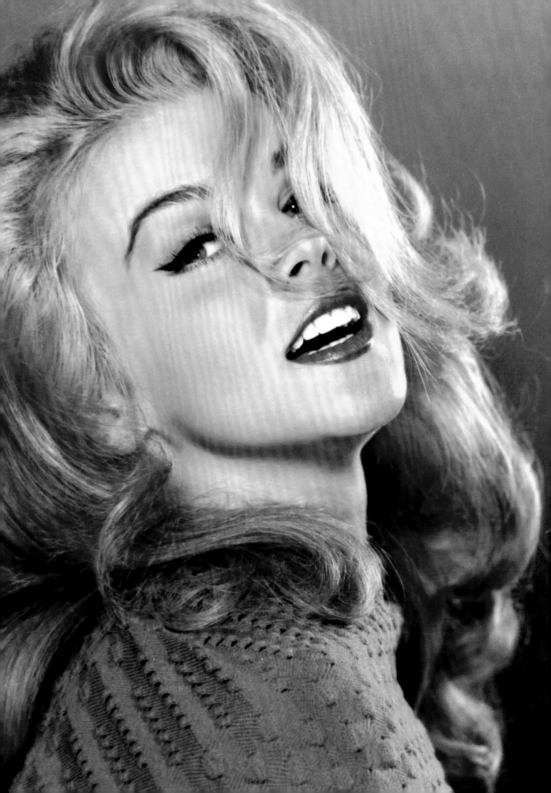

# THE AFRO

★ I can't discuss the hair of the 1960s and not mention one of my favorite styles of all time, the Afro. I loved it back in the day, and I love it now. In the 1960s, many black women who previously wore wigs or straightened their hair decided to cut their hair short and wear it natural as a political statement. I'm for the Afro all the way, at any length, especially today. When Viola Davis stopped wearing wigs and showed up on the red carpet unexpectedly with natural hair, I was cheering for her because it looked stunning. (While her wigs also looked great, there's just something about natural hair and Afros that I adore even more.)

Though the Afro certainly had its heyday in the 1960s and 1970s, many gorgeous women still wear it beautifully today.

Women in the early 1960s either grew out their fifties bouffant into a beehive style or cut it into a shoulder- or ear-length bob that they flipped out at the ends. Bangs were optional but blunt (and a great way to mask a large forehead). Many stars today emulate styles popularized in the 1960s. Vidal Sassoon created a short, blunt bob similar to what the stars are wearing now, and stars like Mia Farrow and Twiggy wore even shorter, blunt cuts—similar to Halle Berry and Anne Hathaway's short locks.

Though most of this era's bouffant styles will make you look like Peg Bundy, stars like Michelle Williams and Zooey Deschanel take inspiration from this era by wearing natural waves with some structure. This can be a great look for women who have some natural wave to their hair, or those who can fake it by using loose rollers. Be careful when styling this, because if your hair looks stiff or super-styled, it won't have the same natural, effortless effect.

The makeup of the sixties is surprisingly straightforward. At the beginning, makeup was very dramatic—to match the huge hair—but later on, the looks were more natural.

If you want to achieve a sixties look with your makeup, decide if you're going early (mod, beehive) or late (hippie, looser). To mimic the early sixties, it's best to go light on your lips and dark with your eyes, and amp up the However, if you're going for a later sixties style, go light on the makeup or don't wear any at all.

# 1970s: *Liberating Beauty*

THE 1970S CONTINUED THE TRENDS of the late 1960s, with nearly everyone sporting long, natural, flowing locks. Unlike previous decades, virtually no styling products were used.

Very little makeup was worn either. Women might moisturize with lip balm or gloss and wear a touch of mascara, but that was all. Makeup was an anti-feminist hallmark and, as such, it simply wasn't fashionable to wear any.

But not everyone in the 1970s was a hippie. Punk began later in the decade by people tired of free love and sit-ins. The punk look combines dark clothes (often black leather) with chunky accessories and heavy makeup. Contrary to its anti-beauty message—or maybe because of it—punk is a timeless style that isn't trendy but is always in style—a true anti-trend.

In the mid-1970s, disco joined punk in contrast to hippie style, introducing the idea of day and night styling. In the daytime, women would wear natural hairstyles and very little makeup—just white eyeliner (which makes the eye appear bigger), concealers, mascara, and lip gloss. However, at night, the beauty look was anything but natural.

The makeup worn by a disco queen is remarkably similar to what a drag queen

## WHAT'S THE PURPOSE OF MAKEUP?

★ Do you wear makeup to accentuate your beauty or to hide your flaws? Prior to the 1970s, cosmetics companies focused on how their makeup would accentuate the eye, make the lips look fuller, or draw attention to whatever feature was popular at the time.

However, after the no-makeup looks of the sixties and seventies, cosmetics manufacturers were forced to change marketing strategies. Instead of selling women makeup by promoting natural beauty, the companies marketed products that hid "flaws" instead. Unfortunately, this is still the practice today. Most of us wear makeup to cover whatever we perceive to be our "problems," rather than taking a tip from the leading ladies of the past and using cosmetics to emphasize our best features.

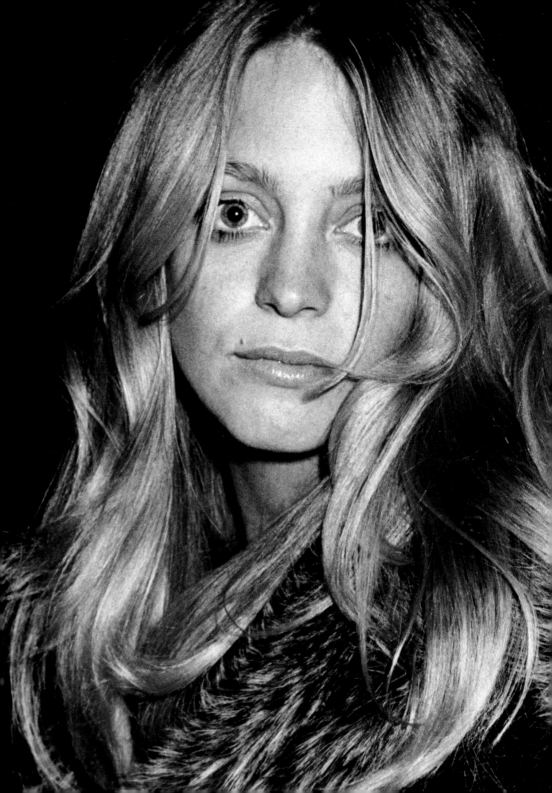

wears today. Both tend to wear heavy metallic eye makeup, sharply define their cheekbones and eyes (using the power of highlighters and eyeliner, respectively), and have glossy lips. Women were disco warriors, and wore their war paint to the club.

Though mimicking the styles of this decade can create a bohemian beauty or magic retro glam, be wary of combining too many elements in one look. It's easy to take one step too far into the seventies and leave your house looking like a hippie lost in time—or worse yet, a drag queen on her way home from a show. No offense to drag queens—I love you!—but no woman wants to look like a man dressed as a woman!

# 1980s: *Drama Queens*

FOR A LONG TIME, the eighties have been the joke decade—the "can you believe we looked like that?" period—and people would never dream of duplicating the styles they wore back then. Though I'm not advocating that you walk out the door in full-on eighties gear, there *are* makeup looks and hairstyles that can be transitioned to fashionably chic today.

In the eighties, thanks to hair products like mousse and gel, women were able to achieve big and bold looks with their hair. From Brooke Shields' voluminous long locks to the multifaceted colors of singer Cyndi Lauper, hair was big, curly, and sculpted.

Perms and coloring were in vogue as well, particularly two-toned and frosted hair. To this day, frosted hair cracks me up! It's your hair, not a cookie.

If you want to embody eighties style, just think the word "more." *More* hair, *more* color, *more* brightness, and most important, *more* makeup. Women essentially painted their makeup on. A pale and striking look became massively popular by the end of the decade, and to achieve that patina women would wear foundation two or three shades lighter than their natural skin tone so their other makeup would pop more.

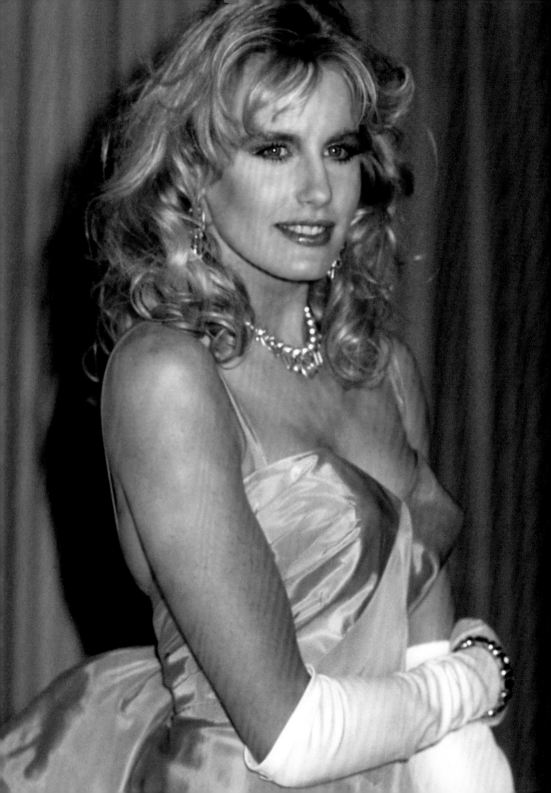

# SUPERMODELS AS BEAUTY ICONS

From the early 1980s until the late 1990s, supermodels took the place of movie stars as beauty and style icons. In the eighties, models like Brooke Shields, Paulina Porizkova, and Christie Brinkley were featured on magazine covers and in tabloids, famously dated and married musicians and movie stars, and were heralded as trendsetters in fashion and in culture.

By contrast, in the 1990s, participating in fashion was seen as vapid or corporate for anyone outside the actual industry, including actors. Being glamorous was seen as "selling out," so major movie stars of this decade, such as Winona Ryder and Drew Barrymore, kept a relatively low-key public profile—or tried to—while supermodels (including the trifecta of Linda Evangelista, Christy Turlington, and Naomi Campbell) reigned supreme as trendsetters.

The disco queens of the seventies had nothing on stylish eighties girls. These ladies wore eye shadow all the way up to their brow, in stark and bright colors like blue and silver. I remember as a young boy watching my sister literally paint on her eye makeup, applying it over and over again so that it would remain as dramatic all day as when she put it on. Once I suggested that she paint her eyelids in a rainbow, not knowing at the time that David Bowie (as Ziggy Stardust) had already done it! To this day, I still wish she had painted her eyes that way, because it would have looked pretty awesome on her.

In addition to crazy eye shadow, matching eyeliner and mascara were used on both top and bottom lids, often "winged" out at the sides to draw an overly dramatic eye. Unless you had naturally thick eyebrows like Brooke Shields, you faked it by penciling more brow in—and created dramatic cheekbones by using blush instead of highlighters.

I remember seeing my older sisters sucking in their cheeks to apply blush. During the eighties, it was fashionable to wear blush purposely in the hollow of the cheek and straight back to the hairline. Shimmery powder was added

# GEORGE'S GUIDE TO
# PLASTIC SURGERY

I'll just come out and say it: I had a nose job. I've always hated my nose. I felt it was bulbous and round and fat and not at all distinguished looking. So in 1994, I started to look into plastic surgery.

First of all, if you're considering plastic surgery, aim for a natural look. You don't want people noticing that you've had work done. Your goal should not be for anyone to notice or ask what you had done. Your goal is for people to simply say, "You look great!" If plastic surgery is done well, that's what will happen.

Second, consider your (actual) age. Many women who have work done in their thirties or forties, trying to look younger, end up looking older than they actually are. I have a way of describing how women who've had bad plastic surgery look: somewhere between the age of thirty-five and sixty-five. It's very disconcerting, to say the least. It's important to be wary of

having major plastic surgery before you are well into your forties, because having work done too early can almost literally knock the life out of your face.

Third, be sure to shop around. The first plastic surgeon I went to—keep in mind, this is before everything was digital—took a Polaroid picture of my face and drew me a new nose with paint. But he also added a stronger chin. I was so taken by this drawing that I was convinced I needed not only a new nose but a new chin too! Luckily, when I went home and told my roommate what I was about to do, she told me I was out of my fucking mind. Those were her exact words—and she was exactly right. I came to my senses immediately and realized that though I wanted a new nose, I already had a chin! I didn't need another one!

The surgeon I went with, Dr. Raj Kanodia, treats his work like it is his art and his patients, the palettes.

He would have never suggested giving me a new chin, because Dr. Kanodia always aims for the most natural look possible. In close to twenty years since I've had my altered nose, only one person has ever been able to tell. (And that was a bitchy queen, so whatever!) Even my mother didn't notice when I first had it done! Granted, I was living in California at the time and she hadn't seen me in months, but still—this is the woman who gave birth to me, and her only comment was that I looked good. That's how superb Raj is with noses! Basically, what plastic surgery did for me was to reshape a feature I hated, which ended up taking off more than a few years and making my overall look much more refreshed and youthful. Well worth it!

But it's important to do your research: Talk to different doctors about their approaches and opinions, and speak with close friends about what you plan to do so that you don't make a spur-of-the-moment, uneducated decision.

Changing your appearance with surgery is a big deal and should be treated that way.

Last but not least, if you think plastic surgery is going to change your life in some big, sudden way, that's not a good reason to do it. Having a new nose or fewer wrinkles won't make Mr. Right appear or bring you a bunch of new friends. And if you have underlying issues about your self-image, be careful about going under the knife, because changing your appearance that way can get out of control quickly or put you in a negative spiral. Let Heidi Pratt from *The Hills* be a warning.

However, if there's something about yourself that you've always disliked, it's OK to fix it—with realistic expectations—because I know, from experience, that it will actually make you happier. Sometimes, making small refinements, which movie stars do all the time, can take a person from being pretty to absolutely stunning.

afterward to make the cheekbones stand out even more. Last but not least, lips in this era were glossy and large; bright colors like fuchsia and orange dominated with traditional reds still lingering a little bit.

For the most part, the makeup and hair of the 1980s was totally overdone and will look even more so if you duplicate it today. However, some of the minor elements—like doing a strong lip and a strong eye simultaneously—*have* come back into fashion.

# 1990s: *Glamour or Grunge*

THANKS TO THE ANTI-ESTABLISHMENT, anti-trend vibe of this decade, there were several hair trends going on at the same time. Popular styles included grunge (looking like you just rolled out of bed with dirty hair), multifaceted hair color and highlights (hello, Manic Panic), stick-straight, center-parted hair like Alicia Silverstone's in *Clueless,* and later on, layered styles like the "Rachel" haircut popularized by Jennifer Aniston on *Friends*. Since multiple styles were trendy, there wasn't so much a standard length as there was a sort of standard vibe for hair.

Whether you had a blunt cut or wispy layers, hair at any length was styled stick straight or barely flipped under or out at the ends. Since that look is hard for most people to achieve, anti-frizz products and straightening irons dominated the market. However, by the end of the 1990s, casual, sun-kissed, tousled hair that looked like you had just returned from a beach took the place of strict style. "Beachy hair" is still on trend today.

Makeup in the 1990s was about more than just your face. Hard Candy nail polish brought in stark colors, and Chanel Vamp popularized black nail polish. On the flip side of the gloomy nails (and the entire grunge aesthetic), body glitter became ridiculously popular by the middle of the decade. The nineties also marked the first time that cosmetic surgery was accessible to the masses. Nose jobs, face-lifts, lip injections, Botox, breast implants, and even tooth whitening

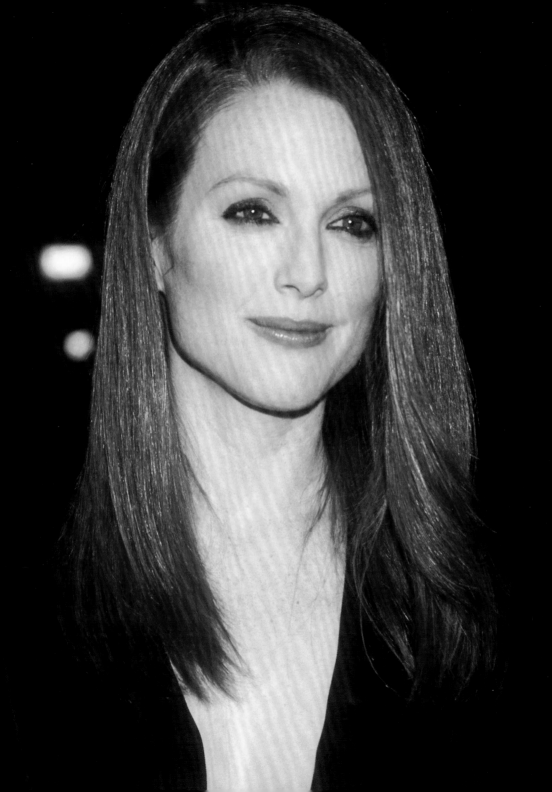

suddenly became affordable options for the general public, instead of just being for aging starlets and trophy wives. But while everything on the body was being plumped, makeup and hair remained minimalist.

Though the decade began with heavy makeup, by the turn of the millennium it was fashionable to wear more natural-looking makeup, which transitioned into today's styles. ★

# ERA MASHUP

★ The same rules that apply to wearing vintage fashion apply to vintage beauty looks. Think of fashioning your hair and makeup just like you would choose an outfit. Combine different trends from various past decades to create a complete, contemporary look that works together and makes you stand out from the crowd.

Truly, anything may go in terms of hair and makeup these days, but be careful not to cross the line. If you copy two bodacious trends from the same over-the-top decade, it will look like you're either a clown headed to a child's birthday party or dressing up as Dee Snider from Twisted Sister.

Whether you copy the hair of Lauren Bacall or the hair of Marlo Thomas at the end of *That Girl,* borrowing from the past in terms of beauty will always work, provided you follow my rule and keep the standout elements of your hair and makeup—or overall beauty look, as we stylists say—limited to two facets. In other words, if you make your hairdo dramatic, it's best to do minimalist makeup except for one standout element, such as dramatic eyes OR killer red lips. On the flip side, if you choose a natural, minimalist, or classic updo with your hair, then you can go all out on your eye makeup and draw from the over-the-top faces of the sixties or eighties.

Remember: Cultivating vintage movie-star style is about the overall presentation, not the timeline. Feel free to copy winning trends from the past that complement your outfit and the overall look you want to achieve—but be wary of copying verbatim any decade, vintage look, or leading lady.

# RISING-STAR
# REMINDERS:

★ The reason stylists call hair and makeup a "beauty look" is that the two are inseparable. If a woman has great hair and overdone makeup, she looks like a hot mess. If a woman has unstyled hair and perfect makeup, she looks disheveled.

★ A bad hairstylist is like a bad boyfriend. If you're not with the right person, then you're wasting time. Get a haircut that suits your face shape, hair texture, and best features, and that also reflects your personality.

★ You can never go wrong emulating the classic hairstyles of the 1940s or the peachy makeup from the 1950s. These styles look great on most women, and are easy to update for a contemporary yet original look. That's why they are my favorite!

★ Your look shouldn't shout from the rafters. Create just two points of interest to stand out in your hair and makeup for a flawless, starlet-like appearance.

★ Vintage hairstyles and makeup tend to look more sophisticated and elegant than the casual styles we wear today.

★ Use a strategy from the past and concentrate on makeup that accentuates your beauty rather than concentrating on "fixes" for your "flaws."

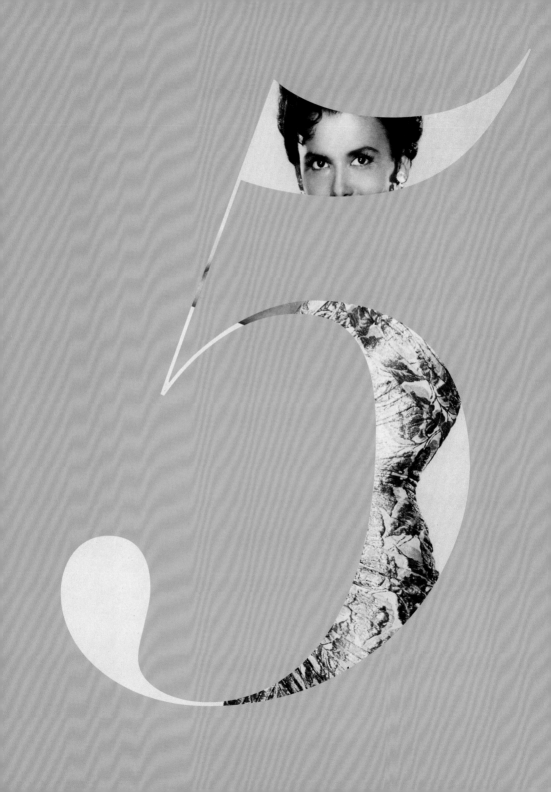

# entertain
*like a*
# movie star

**I**N CLASSIC FILMS, parties of every kind are elegant soirées filled with impeccably dressed men and women enjoying cocktails, meeting new people, and falling in love. Or, in the case of *Breakfast at Tiffany's,* a riotous scene with the hostess plunked down in the middle having a fabulous time, being just as wild as her guests.

As part of being a stylist, I attend *a lot* of parties. Each week, I go to anywhere from four to six parties, from fashion and entertainment-industry affairs to events hosted by friends and family. I've seen the good, the bad, and the ugly when it comes to gatherings. I've been to black-tie events where the music was too loud, there was barely any food, and the room was too dark—as well as low-key soirées where the lighting was perfect, the music ambient, and the food delicious.

I miss the days when everyone knew how to put together an elegant gathering and be a gracious guest. Just fifty or sixty years ago, any woman could put together a nice dinner party—even on the fly—and knew how déclassé it was not to show up after RSVPing yes to an event. But in today's world, entertainment etiquette seems tossed out the window, along with the idea that yoga pants are not just for yoga. (But, they are!)

# Let's Party

JUST AS WITH AN OUTFIT OR HOME DÉCOR, the difference between OK and OMG great for an event is presentation and packaging. By taking into consideration what your guests will expect, want, and need, you'll make a fabulous impression that people will talk about.

In today's world, there are tons of different parties you could potentially have. Whether your event is an informal backyard picnic or a formal wedding reception, most of the same rules about being a generous host and a gracious guest still apply. This isn't a party book, so I'm not going to describe and detail every possible party you could ever have or attend. I will instead concentrate on the two most common parties people (and movie stars) host at home: dinner parties and cocktail parties.

Every party starts with an invitation. When creating an invitation, carefully consider who your guests are and what their lifestyle is like. Be as exact as possible about the date, time, location, dress code, and any special instructions on what you'd like your guests to bring, wear, or consider before coming to your party (including any specifics on directions, parking, or food).

When setting a time for your event, it's crucial to keep in mind what would be appropriate and convenient for your guests' schedule. For instance, if you plan to invite families (both parents and kids), an afternoon event is much more considerate than a party that lasts well into the evening—whereas a party with your young, single friends could be set much later at night.

It's also important to be aware of how long you expect the party to last. Many people make an all-too-common mistake of offering a huge span of time for their parties, such as 7:00 p.m. to 2:00 a.m. That's a crazy amount of time!

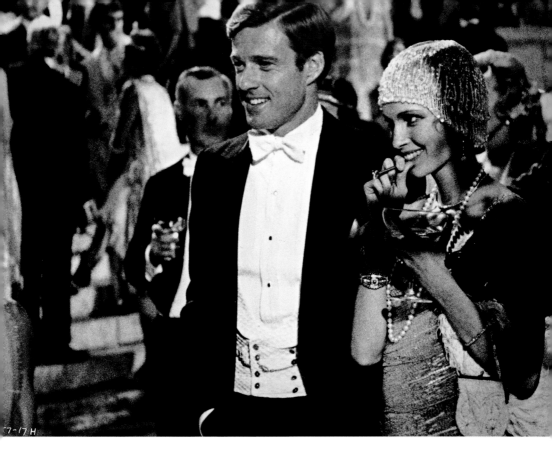

The hosts are trying to be flexible, but often this ends up being a mistake. If you have a large window for the party, guests have no idea when others will arrive. No one wants to be at a party alone!

Narrowing the window of time for your party to three or four hours encourages guests to show up around the same time as one another—creating a more populated and fun party—and encourages your guests to reserve their entire evening for your event.

The main difference between a dinner party and a cocktail party is that a full dinner is served at the former, whereas a cocktail party is exactly that: cocktails with snacks or hors d'oeuvres. A hard-and-fast rule of mine is that snacks must be served at any soirée. I think it's rude to invite people over without food being offered (perhaps because I'm Greek and we love food).

# A NOTE ABOUT
# THE TIME

★ Be wary of the dinner hour unless you're hosting an actual dinner party. Part of being a great host is making the event as easy to attend as possible for your guests. In addition to being mindful about what you're planning to serve for food—because every party needs nosh—schedule your event so that guests will clearly know whether to eat afterward or beforehand. If you plan on serving "heavy hors d'oeuvres" or something equivalent to a meal, say so on the invitation. Keep in mind that the dinner "hour" takes place roughly between 7:00 and 9:00 p.m., though this varies upon your age, lifestyle, and where you live.

Once again, it's important to consider who will be attending and when they typically eat. If you're not serving hearty food, it's safest to schedule the party to take place either before or after the dinner hour. In places like New York and Los Angeles, where dinner is typically served between 7:30 and 8:30 p.m., starting a party at 6:00 or at 9:00 is wise; elsewhere, earlier or later may be better.

What you are planning to serve should be included on the invitation. Telling your guests what to expect regarding food makes your party easier to schedule and more comfortable to attend. This applies to location as well—if your home or the venue is tricky to find, has limited parking, or could otherwise inconvenience your guests, be sure to let them know. For instance, I've been to a few events held at glorious estates or amazing parks. Sure, that sounds great, but not if you're a woman in heels! The beautiful surroundings are contrasted with ladies trying to pull their stilettos out of the grass with each step, making the event much less elegant and affecting the entire mood of the party. You're not exactly going to be cheery if you just ruined a pair of Louboutins or twisted your ankle. In that particular case, the invitation should have included a warning that the event would take place on grass, thus tipping off women to wear wedges or flats, not stiletto heels. This rule particularly applies to outdoor or beach weddings.

Essentially, a host wants to avoid anything at his or her party that could even remotely create frustration or confusion, whether it's a guest getting lost, not being able to find parking, or wearing the wrong shoes. At parties, just as in life, the first impression is what lasts.

Once you have the party's venue, timing, and special considerations for location on the invitation, you should consider the attire for the event. If you don't specify a certain type of attire, guests will come as casual or as elegant as they want (which can be good or bad, depending on your guest list!).

## Répondez s'il vous plaît

IN THE PAST, it was standard to include a dress code and a RSVP date on any invitation—and although many people have let this part of etiquette go, I think we should work to bring it back. If you get an invitation with an RSVP, respond immediately (or at the very least, within a day or two—anything beyond that is rude). It's not only kind to the host—who has an idea of what she wants her event to be like, and needs to know how many people are coming—but makes every event more fun to get ready for and attend.

# If You Are Hosting . . .

AFTER INVITATIONS FOR YOUR PARTY ARE SENT, the prep work begins. In addition to thoroughly cleaning your home (or paying a cleaning service to do it), you should create a shopping list for everything you need. If it's your first time hosting a party or you haven't entertained in a while, it could be helpful to visit a home-goods store. As I've mentioned, great design is available at every price point, and that's especially true when it comes to dishes, flatware, and glasses for entertaining. Places like IKEA, West Elm, HomeGoods, CB2, and many other stores offer dishes for entertaining that are surprisingly inexpensive. There's no need to spend tons of money on entertaining ware, whether it's china or wineglasses, because there are less expensive options—and frankly, not many of us need fancy goblets or multiple china patterns.

A few years ago I bought about forty water goblets and medium-sized glasses (which work for highball cocktails and wine) at IKEA for around thirty dollars and stored them in a not-so-reachable part of my kitchen. Whenever I host a party, I get out a ladder, pull all those glasses out, and use them! The glasses work for every kind of drink, so I don't have to fetch different kinds of glasses for various guests, and because of how cheap they were, I don't worry if any of them break. After the party, I wash the glasses in the dishwasher, haul out the ladder again, and put them back in the cabinet. Chic and cheap!

At a certain point in your life, using plastic becomes tacky, especially since party glasses have become so inexpensive. My rule is that you shouldn't use cheap plastic at a party unless it's part of the theme and used with irony.

When I receive a plastic cup at a party, I instantly receive the message that the host does not care. He doesn't want to have to deal with having to get me a glass, clean up afterward, or present his home in an elegant way. And while that's fine for some people, it certainly isn't movie-star chic. So if you want to be elegant and entertain like a starlet, ditch the plastic and get some glasses!

In advance of a scheduled party, it's always handy to have a wide variety of sodas, liquors, wine, and beer available for your guests. Though you can assume many people will bring beverages to your party, it's best to be prepared.

In addition to alcohol, having food on hand is key. Stores like Trader Joe's or Costco are great resources for inexpensive bites that can be ready in a flash. Any appetizer that can be popped in the microwave or oven or can otherwise be made and presented within a fifteen-minute window is ideal for entertaining. Crudités, nuts, olives, cheeses, crackers, and dips are all wise choices for parties. Fresh is always best, but in a pinch, there are frozen options.

On long fashion shoots, we often have craft-table service all day. So not only are there snacks on hand, there are also appetizers being passed. Once, I had a chicken satay so delicious that I had to ask where the caterer got it from—and the server discreetly whispered to me, "Don't tell anyone, but it's from Costco!" This was another instance that showed how, just as with fashion, chic can be cheap when it comes to party food.

# THE
# WOW FACTOR

★ A "party" can suddenly appear out of nowhere. You're out with friends and the bar closes, or you decide to go somewhere quieter to talk with your best friends, book club, or a date. If you follow my instructions and prep your kitchen and bar beforehand, you'll be able to confidently offer up your home as a venue—and voilà, instant party!

Inviting guests to your home unexpectedly and then having everything they desire—a few different drink options and hot appetizers ready to pop into the oven or microwave—will really make an impression. You'll be seen as an exceptional hostess prepared for everything, because you are.

The most convenient time to make sure your kitchen and bar are prepped for an unexpected party is when you're preparing for an actual scheduled event. But even if you don't have a party coming up, it's never the wrong time to buy a few bottles, store some mixers, and go a little crazy in the freezer aisle at Trader Joe's. After all, tomorrow night might present an opportunity for an impromptu party!

Presentation is all about the packaging, so never serve dips or appetizers in their original containers. This is what entertaining dishes are for! Create a central area for food and drinks (usually situated in or near the kitchen) with some additional snacks placed around the other areas you want guests to be in. It's nice to have different dishes at varying heights on a table. Offering snacks in a few small bowls—that you refill when empty—is more classy than putting everything you have in a giant bowl. There's always something a little gross about a giant bowl of nuts or vat of olives. If you *have* to use a big container for some reason, provide tongs or a serving spoon in order to avoid everyone's fingers touching the food.

Once you have the food and the drinks figured out, it's time to set the mood. Lighting is key! For any party, but especially cocktail and dinner parties, you want a sexy nightclub vibe—your home shouldn't look grocery-store bright. I can't tell you how many chic celebrity homes I go to where the lights are turned up rather than down—such an easily avoided mistake! Your home, especially when you are throwing a party, is a place to relax—not the surface of the sun. You wouldn't stay at a bar or restaurant that had bright lights inside, would you? Of course not! I have the same philosophy for homes.

As a general rule, aim for at least three sources of lighting in every room (minus the kitchen, unless you have an open-plan apartment or home). Some of you might be thinking: How do I get that many lights? It's actually very easy.

Side lighting—such as art lighting or wall sconces—is really the best for creating a relaxing, cozy mood in a home. Floor lamps and table lamps are also great soft sources of light. Many lamps have three-way switches so you can control the amount of light, though attaching dimmers to lamps is another easy option. It's also chic—and very French—to have a bit of gold foil inside a lampshade, which creates a golden glow throughout the room.

The very best thing I ever bought for my home is a remote control for a pair of lamps I have. With just one click of a button, both lights come on—and if you hold the button down, the light can be brighter or dimmer in a second! That, coupled with the ability to control my sound system with my iPhone, makes me feel like I'm living in Rock Hudson's lair from a Doris Day movie.

If you don't have the budget to buy all-new lamps, adding candlelight is the most inexpensive way to create a romantic, flattering glow for any room. Everyone loves candlelight! It will make any occasion feel special. Candlelight is the most forgiving light possible. It hides scuffs on the wall, makes everyone appear younger and more attractive, and is inexpensive to buy and replace. You can buy a hundred votive candles and small glass holders for a few dollars. For a fun, eclectic look, buy a bunch of different colors and styles; votive holders don't have to match. Be sure to also buy a long lighter; it's the easiest and safest way to light a bunch of candles.

Candlelight can really transform a space. Once, I went to a party at this beautiful lounge in Los Angeles, which had gorgeous velvet-covered banquettes, perfectly painted dark gray walls, polished old-fashioned wood floors, and tons of candlelight. I loved the décor so much that I had to go back—but

# GOING OUT FOR YOUR PARTY

Many of my friends book restaurants and bars as party venues, especially for birthdays and big occasions. If you decide to host a party outside your home, be sure to indicate whether guests will have to pay for drinks (cash bar or not), and if so, be considerate about how much a drink costs. For instance, going to a bar that charges fifteen dollars per drink is rude if your guests tend to be on a tight budget, whereas going to that same bar later on in life, when your friends have careers that pay well, is totally appropriate.

It's considerate and kind to make sure the bar or restaurant you choose is affordable for everyone who will be attending. There are great bar and restaurant options at every price point. Many establishments will allow you to come up with a couple of specialty cocktails or types of drinks you'll provide (with anything other than those drinks being paid for by guests). You can also arrange for an open bar during the first hour of a party and then switch to a cash bar for the rest of the evening. There's nothing wrong with either of those options, unless everyone knows that you can afford to pay for everything—then you're just being cheap.

A big advantage to having a party outside your home is that other people are doing the work for you, pouring drinks, and serving food. However, leaving the host duties to others comes with different responsibilities for you, like making sure that your contract or agreement with the venue covers exactly what you want and what you expect your guests to want or need. If you decide to do an open bar for an hour or only pay for certain drinks, you should specify in advance the maximum dollar amount you want to spend so there are no surprises. It's also important that if the service becomes lackluster at any point, as the actual host of the party you shouldn't hesitate to take the manager or waiters aside to quietly correct it. After all, you're the customer!

when I returned it was daytime. The lounge had a totally different feel, and it was not good. In bright light, this place was disgusting! The velvet was filthy, the walls were grimy, and the floors were covered in all sorts of gross stuff. The candlelight had made a massive difference in how everyone saw the space—

# GEORGE'S GUIDE TO ATTIRE

Because most people don't attend a ton of formal events—and I do—friends and fans often ask me to define types of attire. Since every movie star worth her salt knows what each of these terms mean, so should you.

## Business Casual

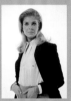

This depends on what your business is, but typically it's either what you wear to work on an average day or what you would wear to a nice (but not Michelin-starred) restaurant on a date. For women (and men), dressy jeans with a great blazer is perfect. In many creative fields, this is often a mix of casual and cocktail looks.

## Casual

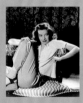

Pretty much anything goes. This is really defined by your own personal style, but when I see "casual attire" on an invite, I wear the same outfit as I would to drinks with a colleague or friend or date I want to impress. This outfit should be more fashionable and festive than your average Tuesday, but it's definitely not couture.

## Semiformal

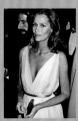

This can vary, but semiformal or informal is more fancy than business casual but less flashy than cocktail attire. (If you're unsure, overdress.) Semiformal for men is typically a dark evening suit with a tie—you can spruce up any man's outfit with a tie—and women typically wear knee-length dresses or simplistic gowns. Semiformal dresses for women are not nearly as sparkly, fancy, or short as cocktail dresses. Think simple and elegant.

## Cocktail Attire

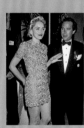

Cocktail wear is the middle ground between casual and formalwear. It has some elements of formality, but it's not black tie. For women, this is a cocktail-length or mini-length dress with great shoes and accessories. Men could wear a casual suit, or better yet, a tailored blazer with a tie and dark jeans. When I go to a party in cocktail attire, I almost always wear a necktie. It instantly dresses up any man's look. Women should feel free to be sparkly when cocktail attire is requested.

## Black Tie

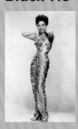

This is formalwear, plain and simple. Men should wear a tuxedo, and women should wear a gown or a very dressy and embellished tea-length dress. Women should not wear a minidress, or even a cocktail dress, no matter how embellished or "dressy" the piece is.

## Adjective Attire

Where attire gets tricky is when people add words to the traditional definitions. For instance, "creative black tie" means that guests are invited and expected to have fun with their fashion. For men, creative black tie can get a little hokey, but typically I wear a tuxedo jacket with a white shirt, black tie, jeans, and nice black shoes. Women should go all out with their dresses. Most often, though, I see the word "festive" added to the dress code. Ahem, you're automatically going to be festively dressed—it's a party! But this really means that the hosts are asking you to put extra effort into your outfit so their event is more of a "to do" and—dare I say it—festive.

When a host or hostess (or you) adds other words to standard attire definitions, such as "beach formal," it's awkward for guests because the dress code isn't defined. As a host, it's best to stick with the terms people know or can Google. Otherwise, you risk people dressing every which way or having to answer a zillion questions about what people should wear. On the other hand, if you receive an invitation with an odd dress code, it's safest to follow the main term (i.e., the "formal" in "beach formal") or ask your host what he or she will be wearing. In my opinion, invitations should be clear enough so you don't have to ask your host what to wear, but it's not a perfect world!

One last word about attire: Optional is not an option. Either it's black tie or it's not. As a host, either you tell your guests what to wear or you don't. Adding the word "optional" or "preferred" after a dress code is a waste of time, because it's a halfway response. It's like saying "RSVP Optional" or "RSVP Preferred"—do you need to know if people are coming or not? Though it may seem rude to "require" your guests to wear a certain kind of clothing, it's really not. If you want your event to be formal, specify that the dress code is formal or black tie. If you don't care, then you don't care. Ultimately, you're the host, and it's your party, so you determine what you want the style of attire to be. Period.

because the dim lighting hid all its flaws. Candles (and to some extent, dimmer lighting overall) can do the same for your home.

In addition to the right lighting, music is also important. It should be at a volume level where people are aware of it and can hear it, but not so loud you have to shout over it. It's easy to create playlists using online services like Spotify, Pandora, and Rdio or the "Genius" tool on iTunes. Pick a song you love that captures the mood of your party, and there will be a way to start a playlist based off that song. Voilà, instant DJ! You don't necessarily need to hire someone to have great music at your party. All you need is a computer, tablet, or mp3 player.

It's important to figure out what music you're playing a day or two in advance, so you can make sure the playlist you've created "builds"—from a mellow start to a more crazy or beat-heavy mix later on—just like your party will.

An hour or two before the party starts, set the scene: Get the music cued up, set out the room-temp food and drinks, and pour yourself a cocktail before your guests arrive.

# Party Time

ONCE YOUR GUESTS BEGIN ARRIVING, the show is on! The most important thing you can do when guests walk in the door is to get the drinks flowing. Whether you imbibe or not, we are adults, and alcohol is fun. If your guests partake, get them a drink immediately. If they don't, get them a nonalcoholic beverage immediately. Everything in moderation, of course, but get your guests drinking!

If you tend to feel overwhelmed by your host duties and serving alcohol at the same time, feel free to hire a bartender. It's often well worth the cost to have someone in charge of mixing and serving drinks to your guests so you can actually enjoy your own party.

Organically, most parties tend to cluster around where the food and drinks are—typically in the kitchen. At a cocktail party, people will sit wherever there's a seat available—but most people will expect to stand.

That's why most of the food for a cocktail party should be appetizers, hors d'oeuvres, or finger food—anything that can be either held in one hand or eaten off a small plate. In fact, appetizers—particularly passed appetizers—should be eatable in one bite. That not only avoids the juggling act people do when they are holding both a drink and an appetizer in their hands, but it also avoids any potential mess that comes from that juggling act not being completely perfect.

Again, it's important to keep your guests in mind. If you know that some guests have been on their feet all day at work or are older, you'll want to have more seating. If your guests are young or sat around in an office or at home all day, just a few seats will be fine.

There will always be guests who know each other—these are your friends, after all—and some who don't. When introducing guests who don't know each other, it's important to indicate their relationship status. For instance, rather than introducing a married couple simply as "my friends," you should introduce them as "my friend Ben and his wife, Sarah" or "my friend Stephen and his partner, Dave" (depending on sexuality, obviously). Be sure to cover your bases, so you can avoid awkward situations!

If I think my guests might have something in common professionally or personally, I would introduce them and be sure to mention that. For instance, I could introduce a magazine editor friend to a photographer I think she would enjoy working with. I think the best professional connections start with clicking socially. Even hobbies or a common background—both of you love biking or are from New York—can give your guests something extra to talk about (in addition to your fabulous party). Just be sure to make these introductions as nonchalant as you can. It's not chic to make your guests feel like they're being "worked" or that, worse yet, someone is only talking to them to "network." (I have to admit a big part of my business is done while entertaining, and I often get clients by meeting them at a party. But I don't try to sell myself or be

# DINNER PARTY DOS

⭐ Though most of the rules are the same for cocktail and dinner parties, the latter has a few special caveats. If you're planning a dinner party, you need to make sure that there is enough seating for all the guests who have RSVPed or that you expect to come, whether those guests will be seated at your dining table or will be eating from their laps throughout your space. If you're serving a buffet-style dinner, you should immaculately set the table and create a central location close by for food and drinks, with a clear path for the guests to follow (so that serving is quick and easy, not confusing).

If you are doing a seated dinner party, I suggest using place cards and separating dates and friends. Mixing couples, singles, and people who don't know each other encourages conversation among the whole table rather than within twos and threes seated next to each other.

Personally, I love dinner parties, but I think hosting a seated dinner all by yourself can be difficult. If you want to be the chef at your dinner party, a buffet-style event may be more manageable, though you can certainly hire a personal chef or caterers and waiters for the evening to make your seated dinner a truly special occasion. I used to think hiring a personal chef was expensive—but was surprised to find out that many are completely affordable and often are cheaper than taking your friends out to a restaurant.

disingenuous. I simply talk to interesting people, and if they want to hire me, great! But I don't try to work the person I'm with, or network just for the sake of networking. And if I feel like I'm on the receiving end of someone trying to do either of those things, I find a way to end that conversation!)

Some people are great at making new friends and starting conversations with strangers, while others simply aren't. By paying attention and gauging your guests' personalities and comfort levels, you can match one with the other (or pair extroverted people together) to make sure conversation gets rolling.

If you have a mix of people who know and don't know each other, it can help to limit the space that the party is in. The most fun parties I've ever hosted or been to have always been a teeny bit overcrowded. You can have a number of people in a smaller space and have the party feel popular, whereas that same number of people in a large area can feel sparse and not as fun. Even though I love my house, I sort of miss my one-bedroom apartment sometimes, because the parties I had there had a more intimate feeling.

Last but not least, don't be afraid to hire some help. Valets for parking, bartenders for drinks, and servers for food can often be well worth the money! Whether it's a friend serving as cohost or a cute guy serving up drinks, having a bit of assistance can often make the party more fun for your guests and, more important, for you! As a host, you work hard putting a soirée together, and it should be a blast for you as well. If you aren't having any fun at your own party, then guests won't be either. It also helps give the impression that your home is a chic, sexy spot. And remember—always have the number for a cab service at the ready in case some of your guests enjoy your party a little too much . . .

# Be a Gracious Guest

ON THE FLIP SIDE, being a guest tends to be much easier than being a host. First of all, your duties are rather limited. You simply have to show up when you say you will, make sure to bring a hostess gift— and above all else, be utterly charming!

Don't bring your bad mood to a party. About fifteen years ago, I attended a party when I felt really glum—so glum I didn't even try to hide it! When I made a comment to an older friend about my mood, he gave me the best advice for parties ever: Show up in a great mood, or stay home! It's a party; no one wants to hear it—and if you're a constant downer, you won't be invited back!

So leave the stressful work at the office, and the drama at home. It's tough to leave for a party in a blah mood, but I find that once you actually get there, it's an instant mood changer because it's a party! (Also, a shot of vodka on your way out the door never hurts.)

Different parties require different things. If it's a dinner party—especially seated—if you RSVPed yes, your butt had better be there. For a cocktail or informal party, the RSVP (if there is one) is a little less strict. However, you should be as considerate as a guest as you would be as a host. So if you say you will be there, show up—or let your host know why you can't be (and the excuse had better be good). If you don't know for sure, say that. If you can't attend, send regrets.

When you do attend the party, be sure to bring along a hostess gift as a thank-you for being invited. Liquor or wine is always a safe choice, especially since the host or hostess may end up needing—and using—it that very evening! It's fine to put the bottle in a gift bag, but I find wrapping a hostess gift to be wasteful and completely unnecessary. When you arrive at the party, the first thing you should do is to find your host or hostess and present them with the bottle. Get the credit you're due for being a gracious guest by saying hi and making sure the host knows you brought something. If you don't want to bring alcohol, a scented candle or a bouquet of flowers is completely appropriate. (Essentially, any universally liked gift is OK.)

If you are a close friend of the host or hostess, it's very kind and considerate to send her or him a message on the day of the party asking if there's anything specific you can bring. Often, the hostess will know what might be missing from her kitchen—or have an idea of which liquor might be the first to run dry. Saving the host's day can be as simple as picking up some limes or a bag of ice on your way over. It's so easy for you, and it will take a huge load off the host's shoulders.

When it's time to leave, consider the scope and scale of the event. If it's a big party, then it's totally OK to take what is called a French exit by Americans, an English exit by the French, and an Irish good-bye by everyone—that is, to slip out without saying good-bye. You don't want to attract attention or show that people are leaving the party (because it could encourage others to leave), but you can still thank the host the next day by sending a quick note or e-mail. On the other hand, if the party is small you should be sure to thank and say good-bye to your host. If you are a gracious and charming guest, you are sure to be invited back! ★

# RISING-STAR
## REMINDERS:

★ When hosting a party, be as specific as possible on the invitations. In addition to basics like location, time, and attire, be sure to include any special considerations guests need to know.

★ Timing is everything! Be sure that the window of time for your party is reasonable and doesn't conflict with the dinner hour unless you are serving dinner or food equivalent to a meal.

★ When hosting a party at your home, DIM THE LIGHTS!

★ Plastic glasses and paper plates are for frat boys. Find and buy inexpensive glasses, plates, and serving ware for entertaining.

★ Build up your bar and stock your freezer with easy drinks and oven-ready appetizers so you can host impromptu parties!

★ If you want to enjoy your party, hire some help.

★ It's easy to be a gracious guest by flipping the script: Think about what your host or hostess could need, and bring it! Every party needs more ice, and more wine. Period.

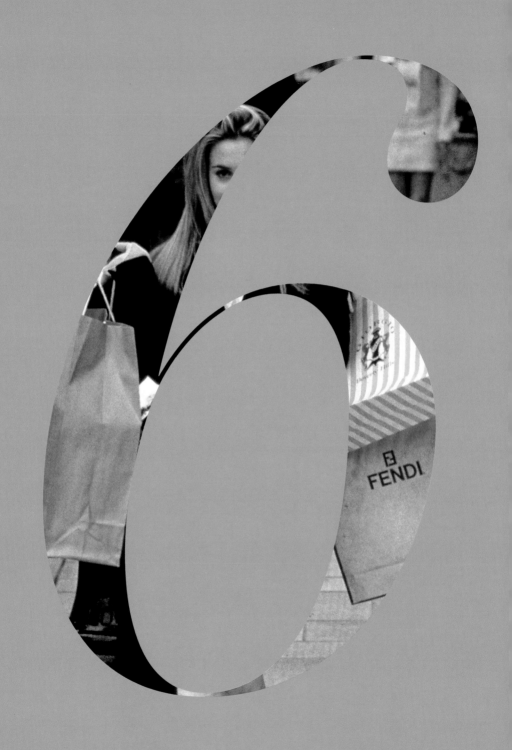

# life's little
# *luxuries*
## *where to save and*
## *where to splurge*

**P**EOPLE LIKE LUXURY. It's nice to feel pampered, to enjoy quality, to wear nicely designed clothes, and, ultimately, feel special. For you, luxury could be as inexpensive as that five-dollar full-fat latte you rarely get. Or it could be investing in a three-hundred-dollar Diane von Furstenberg wrap dress or a really plush cashmere scarf. For me, it was buying my Dolce & Gabbana leather jacket. Yes, it was pricey, but I knew, both from having worn Dolce before and from the quality of the leather, that it would fit me perfectly and last forever. So I splurged—without regret, then and now. Luxury isn't as much about cost as how it makes you feel. Some people can buy a four-dollar cup of organic coffee and enjoy that just as much as I enjoy my Dolce jacket every time I put it on.

It doesn't matter much what you splurge on. But it's really important to choose your luxuries wisely—especially when it comes to your wardrobe. It's

# BE PREPARED

Before you buy anything—splurge or not—it's important to know what you need and what you want (and to be able to tell the difference!). If you've followed the advice in Chapter 1 and have cleaned out your closet and streamlined your wardrobe, you are ready. But if you skipped over that part or thought "I'll do that later" when you read it, go visit your closet before spending any money. Seriously, go figure out what your wardrobe basics are, what you tend to wear or want, and what your closet needs! Movie stars are not procrastinators—especially about their appearance—so put down the book already and get to work!

not smart to spend a ton of money on pieces that will go out of style quickly or that you will tire of, that everyone else will be wearing, or that simply don't fit your lifestyle.

An important part of movie-star style is spending your money wisely and being sure to curate your splurges and saves just as carefully as you curate your closet and home décor. Though the individual decisions about what you should spend and save on are super-personal, I've found in working with clients one-on-one that most people will be wise to save money on certain items of clothing.

There are five items of clothing you can always buy cheaply and still look chic. The two that should be obvious are casual shirts (T-shirts, tank tops, camisoles) and costume jewelry. There's no need to spend one hundred dollars on a T-shirt. American Apparel, Gap, and H&M have nice basics that won't bust your budget. Don't waste your paycheck on a label—no one is going to see it or be able to tell anyway (unless you're wearing a logo shirt, which I shouldn't even have to tell you is so not movie-star style). Costume jewelry, as I've told you throughout this book, can be found so inexpensively that it's ridiculous to spend much money on it.

If you have a good eye, you'll be able to spot jewelry at stores like Forever 21 and H&M that looks expensive at cheap prices. While 70 percent of what these stores have on display is a bit cheap, 30 percent mimics high-end pieces. Forever 21 is not just for twenty-one-year-olds—once in a while, you can grab

# LOGO DOS AND DON'TS

Flashing logos is so tacky. I hate it! If you wear a big logo on your clothes, whether it's emblazoned on the front of your T-shirt, the back pocket of your jeans, or in big bold letters on the side of your sunglasses, you're essentially acting like an ad, which is totally déclassé.

My rule with designer logos is easy: If it is ubiuitous or historical, it's fine. The monograms for Louis Vuitton, Gucci, and Goyard are historical, and the iconic double C for Chanel has been around forever, so those are OK. You should still try to buy pieces that use the monogram as a discreet signal, not a blaring bill-board. But made-up monograms or giant logos simply for advertisement (both advertising that you're wearing the brand and for the brand itself) are not OK.

The lesson here: If I can read the brand of your sunglasses, T-shirt, or bag across the street, you need to go shopping. The point of buying designer is for you to enjoy the quality and craftsmanship, not to blare the brand about. If someone comments on how great your sunglasses are (and they will!), then you can tell them who makes them, just like a movie star does on the red carpet.

great finds there for jewelry. It's all about the edit! In fact, I brought a skeptical client there once, and we found awesome earrings that looked exactly like Lanvin for twenty dollars! For more tricks of the trade, check out my advice on page 52 on how to find great costume jewelry at rock-bottom prices.

You should never spend a lot of cash on anything white. I don't care what it is: white linen pants, a white tank top, a white blouse. Eventually it will develop a stain and be ruined. We once featured Jennifer Lopez on *Fashion Police* because she wore head-to-toe cream-colored leather with small stains on her pants. That stain was bound to happen, so I felt bad, but Jennifer should have known better! (Not to mention checked her outfit before she took the stage.) Anyway, Jennifer learned the lesson so you don't have to: Never spend money on white, because you'll end up with stains no matter how careful you are.

Don't spend a ton of money on pants, including jeans. This may come as a surprise, since pants and jeans are such a staple, but you can get great-looking pants inexpensively. However, you do need to make sure that the material of the pants doesn't look cheap (no synthetic sheen), feels nice on your skin (remember, at least 30 percent natural fibers if you must have a blend, but 100 percent is best), and fits your body well. I'd rather wear a pair of pants from Theory than a $1,000 designer pair, because both take the same amount of time to wear out, and both—this is important—have very little resale value. No one wants to buy pants that have already been worn, so it's hard to get any money back if you change your mind after buying a pair, even if the brand is in high demand. It's not only frugal but practical to buy inexpensive pants made of quality material, whether they are jeans or trousers.

Also, it's silly to spend money on shorts. I bet you have shorts ready to be created in your closet right now. We all have pants that we don't like, for whatever reason, that look OK in the crotch and the butt. Those are perfect to alter and make shorter. Just take your trousers to a trusted tailor and have the pants hemmed to whatever length is flattering on your legs. It's even easier—and totally DIY—to turn jeans into shorts. If a pair of jeans you love develops a rip on the thigh, instant shorts! All you need to make the perfect pair of shorts is a good pair of scissors and a pencil (so if you make a mistake it washes right off). Put on the old jeans, use the pencil to mark where you want the hem (aim for longer, because you can always make shorts shorter after you cut, but never longer), take off the jeans, mark a straight line from the original marker line, and voilà! Instant shorts, and you have an extra forty to a hundred dollars in your pocket. Done and done!

It used to be that stylists (including me) would tell clients to invest in expensive shoes, because you simply couldn't find chic, well-made options at lower price points. However, today that's simply no longer true—stylish shoes are available at every price point, from fast-fashion finds at Justfab.com to expensive collections at department stores.

The truth is, women simply need shoes that look expensive from a distance. When you're going out at night, it's usually too dark to notice detail if you're in a nightclub or a bar, and if you are dining, your feet are under the

# THE TRUTH ABOUT JEANS

★ For some reason, it's fashionable at the moment to spend a ton of money on jeans. Though I understand spending money on clothes that make you look great, I simply don't understand the desire to overpay for an item that has equally chic options at lower price points. Just as with T-shirts, there's really no need to pay for a logo or a tag.

I encourage my clients to try on jeans at every store they walk into, and keep an open mind. The most expensive option might not be what looks the best, even if it's designer. Try on every pair of jeans you like twice: once at the store, and once at home. If it looks good at the store, buy it, and if it still looks good at home, keep it!

Since jeans are so hard to fit, any well-made pair that makes you look great is well worth the money and the search, whether you end up with a $20 pair from Old Navy or a $250 pair of J Brands. Be wary of backstitching, because it looks tacky and cheap on any pair of jeans that's not iconic for its backstitching, like Levi's. Once you know which styles and brands fit you best, it will be easy to replace the old with the new, over and over again.

Ultimately, jeans are a staple where it's OK to splurge if you want to, but you shouldn't feel like you have to.

table most of the time. While it's still important to find quality materials (for comfort and to avoid odor), you certainly don't need to buy Louboutins to look like you have expensive taste. If you can afford the latest work of art Prada has on the runway, by all means wear those beauties! But if not, it's possible to find both classic and trendy styles for evening and day at inexpensive price points. (Unfortunately, for men there isn't such a wide variety. Cheap men's shoes still look cheap—so be sure to invest wisely for yourself or for your man.)

Handbags are similar to shoes, in that there are many more options at varying price points than there used to be. But because a bag is still the item to signify status—more than anything else in the fashion world—I think a great bag is splurge-worthy. In fact, if you can splurge on only one item, it should be a quality bag. As I've said before, I don't really understand the concept of the "It" bag (why would any woman want to carry around the exact same bag as every other woman on the street?), but if there's one thing I do understand, it's enjoying luxury. Having a well-crafted designer bag puts you in an exclusive club that signifies you have a certain income and great taste. It's like saying "I'm stylish!" every time you use it. A great bag can also be practical, if it has a shape and size that suit your lifestyle. But let's be honest. We're not thinking practical when it comes to bags, are we? A general rule for me when it comes to bags is that if it suits your personal style and can be worn with a variety of outfits almost every day, then you should buy it. It's a dangerously low bar . . . but a luxurious one!

That said, I still don't think anyone should spend a month's salary or amass debt for the perfect purse. If you don't have the money to buy the bag with cash, or to pay your credit card bill off in full at the end of the billing period or month, then you can't afford the bag (or any luxury item, for that matter) and you should not buy it. Financial prudence, after all, is chic.

At any price point, when buying a bag you should make sure that the stitch-

# LIAR, LIAR, FAKE LV ON FIRE . . .

Many women try to save money by buying counterfeit and I think that's disgusting. Yes, not everyone can afford real Louis Vuitton, Prada, or even Coach. And yes, fakes are much better made than they used to be. And yes, sometimes (though extremely rarely for someone like me) you really can't tell. But those are not my problems with counterfeit. My issue is that you are lying when you sport a fake bag.

If you're a rich lady with a knockoff, you're cheap and a liar. If you're a girl who doesn't have much money and is carrying a counterfeit bag, you're still pretending to be someone you're not. At the end of the day, it's always more fashionable to be who you are—at any price point—than to pretend otherwise.

Let's face it: If you can't afford a $3,000 bag, that's OK because you don't need one. No one needs a $3,000 bag. If you want a quality bag and don't have a ton of money, there are gorgeous bags out there of equal quality with much lower price tags. You'll have a great bag and be unique—that's movie-star chic.

ing looks good, the lining isn't shoddy, and the leather and hardware don't look cheap. Vintage is a great option for bags, though you have to be on the lookout for stains and general wear and tear, since any bag that's been around for decades will probably have some!

While there are tons of inexpensive options for day bags, evening bags are a bit tougher because cheap satin, more often than not, looks cheap. If you need an evening bag and you don't have a substantial budget, try to find a metallic bag. However, if you attend a lot of events, investing in a Swarovski crystal bag is a smart splurge. If you live to be one hundred, you could bring the bag to every event and still hand it down to your grandchildren. If a crystal happens to accidentally fall or get knocked off, the company will repair it for you. (Actually, most designer retailers will repair their bags—so long as you bought the bag relatively recently and the damage isn't too terrible. Even normal wear and tear is mostly free to repair, or at the very least, worth the repair price, considering what you initially paid and the value of the purse.)

Another item that can be either a "save" or a "splurge" (or sometimes both) is a great coat or jacket. If you live in a cooler climate, fashionable outerwear is an easy splurge, whereas if you live in warmer or more temperate climates you might be able to save and buy a more inexpensive coat simply for travel.

I've been very fortunate because designers often gift me clothes to keep. Any time someone asks me what item I would like, I nearly always ask for a coat. In my closet I have a Louis Vuitton coat, a Versace shearling, a Dolce & Gabbana peacoat, a Balmain leather motorcycle jacket, and a variety of outerwear, several from Brooks Brothers Black Fleece—and I live in Los Angeles! I specifically ask for coats because I travel for work all the time to New York and Chicago, where people see coats just as often as they see your outfit. It should come as no surprise that I think it's as important to look impeccable outside as inside.

However, you don't have to buy a designer coat to look fashionable. There are great inexpensive options at H&M and Zara. Vintage coats can be amazing, especially for women—older coats tend to be warmer and are ridiculously inexpensive compared to new coats. (One friend recently found a vintage fur coat for eight dollars at a thrift store!) Many vintage coats from the 1960s look like Marc Jacobs today. Vintage coats are easy to find in good condition, though you may have to search for a while to locate one that fits. (As with vintage blazers, be sure to make sure the coat fits in the shoulders, because cuts were more demure for Grandma's generation than for today.

Keep in mind that vintage coats, and many designer coats, have bracelet sleeves. Dating back to the fifties and sixties, bracelet sleeves were meant to be fashionable—so women could show off their bracelets—and less bulky. There are many stylish ways to wear bracelet sleeves: with bare arms, short or long gloves, long-sleeved shirts, or, of course, with bracelets. In fact, altering a blazer, jacket, coat, or even a sweater to have three-quarter bracelet sleeves can quickly modernize a piece—and is another great way to refresh an older piece in your closet.

Coats are great investment pieces, because the overall style of coats doesn't change very frequently. (And even if it does, a tailor can easily alter a coat stylistically.) If a coat is classic, you can probably wear it for ten years and need only to make simple fixes like reattaching buttons and fixing torn linings. I have a Calvin Klein Collection cashmere topcoat that I got for a steal about fifteen years ago. It's a bit slouchy and just plain comfy, but it was relatively classic then and has been ever since—so I wear it every now and again. But guess what? Now, the oversized look is on trend for men, so I'm ahead of the curve—automatically in style, without having to spend a dime. I'm super-excited to wear it again.

Shopping with a splurge in mind is great. You have to be patient—to find the exact right thing worthy of your money—but if done wisely, it's a great opportunity to enjoy designer brands affordably.

I have to admit that I'm more than a little hooked on shopping at designer boutiques. From the moment you walk into the store, you get treated like royalty. You have great service, get to walk around all day with a Marc Jacobs or Prada shopping bag (don't underestimate how luxurious walking around with that bag feels!), and then go home with a fabulous new item you'll cherish for a

# HOW TO GET
# DESIGNER DEALS

I try not to pay full retail price for anything. My secret is knowing when the fashion seasons begin, end, and transition. If you shop at stores that are transitioning between looks, you can get amazing deals on everything. A savvy shopper not only knows what she's looking for but when to buy it.

There are two great windows to get good deals, and then a few weeks—inside those windows—to get absolutely the best deals. The first window is for spring and summer clothes: If you go anytime in June or July, you'll get a good deal—but if you shop during the last two weeks (or so) in June, and into the first week (or so) in July, you'll get the absolute best deals. The second window happens over the holidays. If you shop anytime between November and January, you're bound to get a good deal. However, if you go right after the new year—say, the first two weeks of January—you'll get the best deals.

Since the idea of "so last season" is dead and gone, it's smart and savvy to shop at the end of each season for what you need and want. If you love an item now, you're probably going to love it in five years. (And if you don't, you need to revisit the earlier chapters about forming your own style instead of following trends!)

Shopping by season is a great way to save. Here is a broad list of when seasons tend to go on sale (though this may fluctuate a bit):

**HOLIDAY ITEMS:** arrive in stores in October and November, on sale in December or January

**PRE-SPRING / RESORTWEAR:** arrives early January, on sale in stores March or April

**SPRING / SUMMER:** arrives in the early spring, on sale starting in June or July

**PRE-FALL:** arrives in the middle of summer, on sale in September and October

**FALL / WINTER:** arrives at the end of summer, on sale in November

Remember: The key to shopping seasonally is timing—and to not let a great deal or trends influence your shopping principles. Look for wearable clothes that you want or need, and which suit your lifestyle. You'll leave stores happy with new clothes and money to spare.

# SHOPPING ONLINE FOR GREAT DEALS (AND NOT-SO-GREAT ONES)

⭐ I know a lot of people who buy designer clothes at gigantic discounts on flash sites like Gilt, HauteLook, and Rue La La. While these sites can offer great deals, there is a lot of fine print involved, including the fact that many items are nonreturnable. I say be wary of any store—either online or bricks-and-mortar—that doesn't have a solid return policy. "A great deal" becomes not so great when you spend money on something that doesn't fit, can't be returned, and won't make back your money on the resale market.

However, that doesn't mean shopping online is a total bust. Department-store websites like Saks or Nordstrom.com can be great, as can online retailers like Net-a-Porter and Shopbop that have solid return policies. You can check out what you like, order a variety of sizes, and try them on in your own home, at your convenience. It's almost like having your very own personal shopper or stylist. This method can be great for people with busy lifestyles who don't have as much time to shop as they would like. But keep in mind that the caveat is the return policy—make sure you can return what you buy. Also, consider the shipping cost—to your home and, if needed, the return—as paying for the time and gas you're saving by shopping online.

Personally, I love shopping at a store. The experience is worth it to me for the effort, and I think you can get just as good, if not better, deals in person. And you'll be able to feel, touch, and try on the clothes—something you can't do on a computer. But, where you shop—what you choose to wear and/or splurge on—is ultimately a personal decision.

long time. But unless you're an heiress or a stylist who gets free stuff like I do, it's tough to shop designer for everything. It's simply not affordable. Or is it?

As with targeting stores at the end of selling seasons, there are ways to get deals on designer clothes. Timing is the same—know when the sales start, and you'll be halfway there. But it's also important to know what to buy when. All the caveats to seasonal shopping apply, but there are a few extra rules based on what point in the sale you're shopping (as well as what you're shopping for).

First markdown: The discount might not be a lot (25 or 30 percent), but this is when you want to buy your basics: shirts, cashmere sweaters, neutral colors, anything that will be useful for everyday life. Knits should totally be bought at first markdown, because quality is hard to find inexpensively. If it qualifies as a "need," you should buy it at first markdown while stock is still offered in your size.

Second markdown: This is where "need" meets "want." If there are neutrals or basics left over that you want (or need), buy them, particularly if you wear a lot of sweaters or blouses or blazers or what-have-you. (If you're going to have to buy them in the next year or two, you might as well buy them now at whatever discount the store is offering.) You could also purchase evening wear, special-occasion, or more special/less everyday items. Depending on your budget, second markdown is a combination of what you want and what you need.

Third markdown: Hallelujah! This is when the awesome deals come in, sometimes up to 70 or even 80 percent off retail. Buy anything that strikes your fancy: cocktail dresses, whimsical fun stuff, things you want but don't need, and extras (coats, shoes, accessories . . .).

I adore getting designer deals, and I just used this method myself. At first markdown, I bought button-down shirts. At second markdown, I bought a suit. And at third markdown, I bought the "fashion" ties and sweaters no one else was buying. At the end of the sale, you'll spot the truly fun stuff that very few people were courageous (or silly) enough to buy at full price.

## Splurge Does Start with S

DESIGNER OR NOT, there are definitely some items everyone should try to splurge on. Lucky for me, these splurges are easy to remember because they all start with the letter S: shoes, special occasion, and suits.

It may seem odd that I say shoes are both a "save" and a "splurge," but, as with handbags, there are different purposes for different kinds of shoes. For normal evening shoes, save money by forgoing designer options and buying at a lower price point. However, for everyday shoes you should splurge.

Whatever your everyday shoe is—it could be a ballet flat, a boot, an oxford, a pump, or something else—it's smart to splurge for quality. If you buy better-made everyday shoes, you won't need to replace the shoe. You'll simply need to replace the sole every now and again. I've had my YSL boots for years. The uppers need a little maintenance (shining, cleaning, etc.), and once in a while the soles need to be redone, both of which a shoe repairperson or cobbler can do in an afternoon.

I also think special-occasion shoes can be a splurge. How many pairs you collect will depend on how many events you typically attend, but I think buying classically styled evening shoes in a variety of colors will eliminate the need to shop for each event that comes up. A pair of strappy sandals, a pair of peep-toes, and a pair of closed-toe heels are all you need to create a go-to shoe closet for special occasions. If you want the full cadre of choices, buy one of each in nude, gold, silver, and black. (Be sure, though, when buying metallic, to get a "medium" shade of silver or gold. Not the brightest, not the dullest.)

For me, special-occasion wear is always a worthy splurge. It never hurts to have an extra cocktail dress at the ready in your closet. If you find a beautiful cocktail dress that fits you like a glove, buy it! You will find a place to wear it, even if there's no event on your calendar the day you find it. Even if you don't attend a ton of events, there are plenty of opportunities (holidays, anniversaries, special date nights, weddings) when a cocktail dress is appropriate and beautiful.

Last but not least, never feel badly about splurging on a suit. Like special-occasion dresses, you may not know where you're going to wear it next when you buy it, but you will wear it. And because suits always need to be tailored, it's tough to find a nice suit inexpensively. The old maxim is true: A cheap suit always looks cheap!

When you buy an expensive (or a good-quality) suit, the store or salesperson makes sure the suit itself works on you by altering it and choosing the right fabric and cut for your body. I can often tell the difference between cheap suiting and more expensive cuts by the fabric (usually silk or wool for women), the inner or lining (it should lay flat), the pattern, if there is one (it should line up at the seams), and by whether it fits the person wearing it.

The primary considerations when shopping for suits are material and construction. Ideally, both the inner and outer material should be made of natural fibers, though it's OK if the inner is artificial. But construction is crucial. To determine how the suit has been put together, ask the salesperson what the "canvas" is (a canvas is the lining between the inner and the outer). If he or she doesn't know, then 99 percent of the time the suit lacks a canvas. That's important because it signals that the suit has been fused (read: glued) together rather than stitched, automatically making it of lesser quality. If you can find and afford it, a suit with stitching is always better than a suit that's been fused.

It's also good to check whether or not the suit is easily wrinkled. Simply crumple up the separates in your hand. If it stays wrinkled after you let it go, don't buy it! You should also double-check that the buttons appear expensive (though these can be replaced), that the buttonholes on the arms actually work (not crucial, but nice), and that

## REMEMBER RESALE

★ Clothing is like a car. As soon as you take it out the door, it's lost a significant amount of its value, whether it's a $10 blouse at H&M or a $10,000 couture dress. But there's one big exception to that: designer bought at a discount. If you buy anything designer or couture at more than, say, 60 percent off, you'll not only get fabulous clothes affordably but also probably be able to recoup your costs later on, when and if you decide to resell that piece. Clothing can be a nice investment, depending on what you buy, when you buy it, and for what price. It may be a splurge now, but it could be a big save later! Just remember, don't buy something just because of the label—that's never worth it.

the lapel on the jacket or blazer rolls instead of being flattened into a sharp crease. Look specifically at the hems and the vents to make sure there aren't any crazy threads hanging (or hems pulling, which is an obvious sign of fusing). And finally, if the fabric is shiny, that's a cheap suit.

Suit separates and accessories can also be a nice splurge. For women, blouses can often be a worthy splurge because the materials blouses tend to be made of, such as silk, are generally better made at higher prices and can often be found on sale. The same applies for day dresses—these can be a splurge or a save depending on the individual dress and what you pair it with. It's very easy, for example, to pair an inexpensive dress with expensive accessories and elevate the entire look.

Belts and watches can also often be a nice splurge. While quality belts can be found at a wide variety of price points, it's important to consider how you are wearing a belt. If it's going to be hidden under a blouse, something inexpensive is totally fine, whereas a corset belt that will be prominent in your outfit might be worth a little extra money. Watches, too, can be a great splurge, because a well-made watch will remain in your collection for a very long time. If you are a businessperson, a quality watch can be part of dressing for the job you want rather than the job you have.

If you're wearing a quality, but not costly, suit with a Cartier, Rolex, Piaget, or Tiffany watch, people will automatically assume that you are successful and wearing expensive clothes head-to-toe even if you're not. Watches are a little like bags in what they say about you, so it can be totally worth it to replace your Swatch with something slightly more elegant.

The same goes for sunglasses. Wearing a chic pair of designer sunglasses (so long as you follow my logo rules and buy something on which the label is relatively discreet) can elevate your entire look, particularly in summer. However, this really depends on your personality. I never lose sunglasses because I wore glasses when I was growing up, and if I lost those, then I was blind! But other people don't have that experience or my personality, and they lose glasses all the time. So it's really up to you. Buying designer sunglasses could be worth your money or be a waste. Or you could buy a mid-level brand that's fashionable and chic, without the label. Just be sure to buy a pair that suits your face and has UV protection. Like so many other items in this chapter, the decision on whether to splurge or to save is up to you. ★

# RISING-STAR REMINDERS:

★ It's not a great deal if it just sits in your closet. Remember to ask yourself, "Where am I wearing this?" before you buy anything, even if it's 99 percent off the original price.

★ Never, ever spend a ton of money on T-shirts, tank tops, camisoles, costume jewelry, *anything white,* or—God forbid—shorts.

★ You have to kiss a lot of frogs before you find the perfect fit, whether searching for a mate or for a pair of well-fitting jeans.

★ It's smart and savvy to shop at the end of each selling season. Buy basics at first markdown, both wants and needs at second markdown, and the quirky fun stuff at third markdown.

★ When shopping a sale at a designer boutique, consider resale value. If you get a great deal, often the resale value will be equal to, or sometimes even more than, what you paid.

★ You can feel justified splurging on special-occasion shoes, handbags, watches, sunglasses . . . just about anything you expect to use and love for years.

★ The definition of luxury is not designer, per se, but how an item makes you feel.

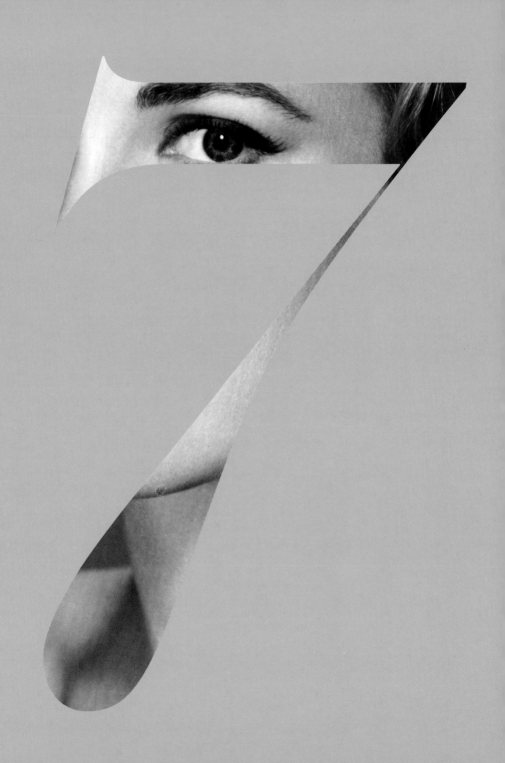

# *be sweet*
## or stay home

H AVING MOVIE-STAR STYLE is more than just wearing a striking outfit, having impeccable home décor, or being able to throw a legendary soirée. In my mind, what makes a person truly glamorous is leaving a lasting, memorable impression of poise, grace, and class.

Of all the leading ladies mentioned in this book, Grace Kelly probably best exemplifies glamorous behavior. For crying out loud, the lady became a friggin' princess! Whether she was the leading lady in a film or doing an interview as the Princess of Monaco, Grace was not only perfectly styled from head to toe but was poised and elegant. It's clear, from interviews and her philanthropy, that she treated people kindly, with respect and dignity. Throughout her lifetime, she anonymously donated money to support emerging artists in the United States, as well as to help orphans in her adopted country of Monaco. When she died after a car accident, her friend and former costar Jimmy Stewart said that Grace was the nicest lady he had ever met, and that "every time I saw her was a holiday of its own."

In today's me-first culture, being inspired by and acting with the same courtesies, manners, and etiquette as movie stars from the past—such as Grace Kelly—will make you stand out like a diamond in the rough. Which you are! In this chapter, I'll share tips on how to act with poise and grace at any occasion, from parties to the office, online, and in person.

# Be Polite

T HE NUMBER-ONE RULE WHEN IT COMES TO BEHAVIOR: Be polite! Acting rude communicates that you don't care about other people, which is selfish and totally not movie-star style. (In my opinion, rudeness is reality-television-star style—which no one should aspire to!)

I suspect most rude behavior comes from people being too busy, being too crazy, or just being in their own world and ignoring everyone else. And though certainly everyone's life gets a bit nuts every now and again, it's never a valid excuse—in my opinion—to be rude or to take that stress out on other people. Period.

"Courtesy" is another word for being polite, though we tend to think of courtesies as actions that we take—like letting an older person take your seat on a bus, for instance, or letting people with children board or disembark a plane before you. Have you ever been on a plane where the cabin crew asks people without connecting flights to wait, so the people who have to make a connection can get off first? I have, and it's always disheartening to see everyone stand up, because you know that the people around you who don't have connections are putting themselves first, when being specifically asked not to. That's the epitome of rude!

In general, being oblivious of people around you—whether it's in the security line at the airport (ahem, everyone should know by now that you have to take off your shoes!), a public place, or in a restaurant—is inconsiderate, impolite, and totally déclassé.

The basic, other than the courtesies I just described, is to say "please" and "thank you" to *everyone,* in almost *any* situation. If someone gives me something—whether it's an awesome gift from a designer or a bartender handing me a martini—I say "thank you." Frankly, I think anyone who is rude, demanding, or condescending to a waiter, bartender, or server is completely gross. On a date, it's a deal-breaker—if a guy does it, we are finished. I don't need to know anything else about you to know that you're a jerk. I find that behavior so unacceptable that I simply don't associate with people like that—and would call out anyone who did.

One of the things I adore about my *Fashion Police* cohost Joan Rivers is that she is lovely, nice, and charming to everyone she meets, particularly the people who wait on her. She says "please" and "thank you"—and *means it.* No matter what, Joan is totally sincere about her manners and showing people respect. So if someone doesn't behave that way, celebrity or not, I think that person is incredibly tacky—and that their momma didn't raise them right! (Mommas, if you are reading this book, teach your kids to say "please" and "thank you"!)

When you get down to it, being polite is really about being considerate of other people. If you cut someone off in traffic (accidentally or only sort of accidentally), raise your hand in the air to acknowledge and apologize for it. If someone around you sneezes, say "God bless you" or "Gesundheit." When you are at the gym, wipe down the machine even if you don't think you actually got sweat on it. And wear deodorant—it may be the gym, but that's no excuse to stink up the place. Be sure to say "excuse me" or "pardon me" when you bump into someone or need to get by. Respect people older than you by addressing them formally: sir, ma'am, miss. It's so simple—there's no reason for rudeness!

It might seem contradictory for me to talk about being polite when my job is to critique people on television. But if you watch *Fashion Police,* you'll notice that I pretty much limit my opinions to the clothes stars are wearing, not the stars themselves. I try not to insult people, both on the show and in real life.

As a general rule, you should never write, say, or otherwise communicate criticism or gossip that you can't tell a person to their face. Did I dislike the dress Halle Berry wore to the 2012 Golden Globes? Yes. Would I tell Halle to her face that I thought the dress was a little tacky? It would probably be a bit nerve-racking or awkward, but if she asked my opinion, I would say that I personally didn't like it and that I think there are better choices for glamorous women such as herself. By the same token, I would tell Jessica Chastain that I adored her dress for the same event, although Joan did not (sorry, Joan!). It's important, whether you're making a public statement on television or not, to be tactful and respectful when talking about other people.

Manners also come into play when you're around other people, whether at a party or in your office. In a strictly social setting—like a party—having great manners and impeccable etiquette is not all that tricky. As I said before in the chapter on entertaining, it's important to become an interesting party guest and conversationalist. Bone up a little on current events, both hard news and pop culture, so you can have an opinion on topics that may come up in conversation.

# Talking Points

THE BIGGEST MISTAKE you can make at parties, or any social setting, really, is to talk too much about yourself. People love people who ask questions, who listen, and allow them to talk about themselves. When you first meet a person, asking questions is always better than telling stories. And be sure to listen! Many people get so caught up in trying to figure out what they'll say next that they actually lose the thread of conversation. There's no need to anticipate conversation, because you will naturally find something to say if you listen carefully and respond authentically.

If you're clicking with whomever you're talking with, the conversation will

# SPEAKING OF TIME . . .

⭐ Try to avoid being late. (Except for fashionably late entrances to parties, which is acceptable.) Being late communicates that not only do you personally not manage your time well but you also don't respect the person's (or people's) time that you're meeting.

I have to admit—I'm terrible at this socially. I always misgauge the time it will take me to do things, and I always try to do "one more thing" before I leave the house (which never ever works!). Since I do believe lateness is incredibly rude, every single time I'm running behind stresses me out to the max, and I apologize profusely when I do arrive. Being late is something I'm working on,

so hopefully by the time you read this book I will have fixed this problem!

Sometimes, though, you can make concessions. A bit of tardiness, especially in cities like Los Angeles (with its heavy traffic), New York (with its random mass transit delays), or Chicago (with its wintery weather), is acceptable. And most of us have friends who are so consistently late that if an event is happening at 8:00 p.m., we tell them 7:00 so there's a chance your group can arrive on time.

But since we're trying to emulate movie-star style, let's all try to be on time. (I promise I'll try!)

eventually arrive at a point where you're asked a question or need to tell a story. This is where having a few go-to stories can be really handy. An "oh my God, I can't believe this happened" tale or funny anecdote is always great for party conversation, particularly if it's generic enough to be suitable for a wide variety of people. But be careful: You don't want to be that person who tells the same story over and over again—so come up with a few to mix in!

Once, my friend Wendy had a great story to share and didn't even know it. One evening she was super-late picking me up for a couple of parties we were planning to attend together. She was delayed because she got sideswiped leaving her driveway! But that wasn't all. The guy who hit her car was a guest at a party nearby and insisted that Wendy join him for a drink. The next thing she knew, Wendy was meeting the host of the party—Arnold Schwarzenegger!

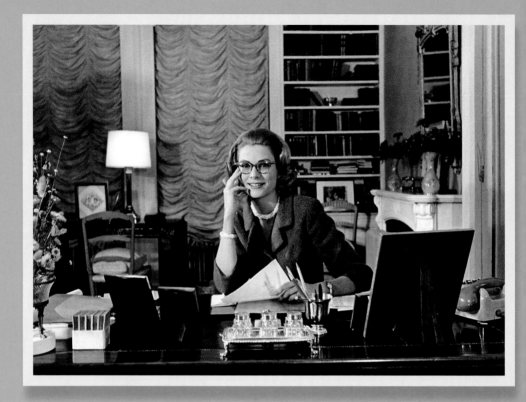

# SAYING THANKS
# THE VINTAGE WAY

Just like taking styles from the past, taking etiquette from the past can be an easy yet super-effective way to demonstrate your sophistication and style. For instance, when a friend invites you to a great party that you really enjoyed, introduces you to a connection that will help your career, offers you genuine personal or professional advice, or gives you a gift (big or small), it's totally appropriate and considerate to send a handwritten thank-you card.

It doesn't have to be fancy—nicely designed cards are available for as low as ninety-nine cents—but it shows your appreciation that takes time and effort. If you find that you are thanking people a lot (such as after a housewarming, wedding, or birthday), investing in personalized stationery can be cheap as well as elegant. Online stationers like Minted, Zazzle, and Paperless Post—along with traditional stationery stores—offer a variety of cards and envelopes that will suit your needs.

When Wendy called me, apologizing profusely, I reassured her by saying, "It's totally fine. Now we have a crazy story to tell tonight!"

So even though both of us were late to parties that night, we had a fun—and totally valid—excuse. Wendy really shouldn't have stressed about it, because her misfortune entertained our hosts, making them completely forget we were tardy!

After all, you're invited out for a reason. Whether it's to a casual gathering of friends or a more formal occasion, hosts invite guests who can contribute. Your contribution may be a great outfit, the ability to make a good drink, your fantastically funny stories, or simply your sociability. If you're lucky to have wealthy friends who invite you to their homes or fancy events, you're being invited not only because you're a friend but also to entertain. We're all entertainers at some point—because everyone wants to have fun, drama-free social experiences. (As I mentioned before, drama is not chic—that's why it's on reality television, not the silver screen!) Being able to converse, mingle with other guests, and get out of conversations with tact are key skills to practice.

## Introducing...

WHETHER IT'S AT A PARTY or in another setting, it's equally as important to properly introduce people as it is to remember people you have been introduced to. If a friend or acquaintance walks up and you don't introduce him or her, it sends the message that the friend or acquaintance is insignificant. If you happen not to remember that person's name, simply introduce the person you were talking to originally, such as "Have you met Sally?" which prompts the new arrival to introduce him- or herself.

Since most of us can't remember every single person we've ever met, it's always safer to say "It's nice to see you" instead of "It's nice to meet you" or "It's nice to see you again" when you are introduced to someone. This is totally a Hollywood trick, because famous people rarely remember everyone they meet—due to the sheer number of people most stars meet! Up until I worked on *Fashion Police*, I could remember whether I had met someone or not. I was

# HOW TO BE
# SORT OF RUDE
# WITHOUT SHOWING IT

Ever been in a totally boring conversation you have no idea how to get out of? You stand there, shifting around, not listening, trying really hard to think of an exit strategy without seeming like a douchebag. This happened to me so many times that I've figured out four proven ways to leave any conversation.

**1. FINISH YOUR DRINK, SO YOU HAVE TO REFILL IT.** "I'm going to get a drink; do you need anything?" is a great way to exit. You'll always see someone you know on the way to the bar, or at the bar itself.

**2. MAKE AN EXCUSE ABOUT FINDING YOUR FRIENDS.** "I haven't seen my friend in a while; want to make sure she's doing OK." Saying that your friend is driving you or only knows a couple of people at the party is a typically safe way to leave the conversation without seeming rude. Often, you will even come off as thoughtful!

**3. HIT THE LOO.** What always works is to excuse yourself to go to the bathroom. No one will question this, ever! It is important to note, though, that if the bathroom is in sight, you should actually go in there, even if it's just to stand inside and check your e-mail while the person finds others to talk to.

**4. BE OBVIOUS WHEN LOOKING FOR OTHERS.** Finally, when you're looking for other people to talk to at a party, make it super-obvious. Traditionally, it's rude to peer over someone's shoulder to see who else is at a soirée, but you can avoid this by saying something like "I love parties, and I love seeing who is here! Don't you?" This changes the focus from "You're not important" to "Let's see who is here," which is much more inclusive and, as a result, less rude!

really proud of that, actually. But now, because I've been meeting so many people, it's getting a little bit blurry. So even I use the "nice to see you" introduction until I remember for sure! For me, all it usually takes is a quick second or a simple reminder, like "I represent so-and-so," "I do the PR for this brand," or "We worked together on this project" to remember how and when I met someone.

The lesson here is that it's better to be vague than to assume and make a mistake. It's incredibly gauche to be the person who doesn't remember anyone—because it communicates, like all rudeness, that you don't care. And because you're glamorous and have movie-star style, you do care!

I'd like to think that I have a pretty awesome memory, but even I don't want to risk it. So unless I know for sure that I've met someone before, I say "It's nice to see you." However, if you have a photographic or otherwise stellar memory, remembering people from your past will make an impression.

For instance, years ago when I was an assistant fashion editor, I met Renée Zellweger. Then I was reintroduced to her several years later. I didn't expect her to remember me, since she is such a big star, but Renée did! At the time, I was flattered and impressed that she knew exactly who I was and when we had met. She left a lasting impression on me, and I could tell from that experience why she is such a big movie star—she's considerate of and nice to everyone.

# Text-tiquette

IN ANY SOCIAL SITUATION, you should limit how much you use—or even check—your phone. A quick text to send directions or tell a friend you're there is OK, as in a quick Foursquare check-in or tweet about the party. Unfortunately, some of us (myself included) live in a world where social media postings are a job requirement. In social or business situations, using your phone to post statuses, tweet, or instagram should happen only once, with the explanation that you're doing it for work (and even in this situation, a quick apology to your friends or guests is nice).

But other than that, put your phone away! I know that I'm at a great party or having an awesome time with my friends when it doesn't even occur to me to check my phone while I'm out. However, if you absolutely need to respond to a text or take a phone call, excuse yourself, walk away, and be sure to apologize when you return. If I'm with a friend or a date who is checking his or her phone all the time, I get offended—because it sends the message that you'd rather spend time with your phone than with me!

While we're on the topic of phones, I really need to say that many people have no idea what's actually appropriate to write in a text, an e-mail, on social media, or all of the above. Texting is not the same as having a conversation. Call me old-fashioned, but I think a text is meant to be a quick note, like passing a note in school.

A call is required when the reason you are reaching out is too complex or urgent for a text. Phone etiquette when calling used to be simple: If the person isn't available when you call, you should leave a voicemail. But I've noticed that many people don't check their voicemail or have a full voicemail box all the time (because they don't check their voicemail . . .). Clearly, these people choose to communicate through texting and e-mail. Since texting is relatively new, so are the etiquette rules about it. Frankly, I don't even know what's the "right" thing to do.

But when it comes to making calls, most people have a missed-call feature on their phones to show that you called them. However—thanks to the butt dial—you should either leave a voicemail or send a follow-up text or e-mail to ensure that the person you called knows that you truly need to speak with him or her.

When you are actually making a call on your phone, be discreet. It's rude to talk on your phone while hanging out with friends or in close quarters with anyone—whether that's at a store or in an elevator. We have all been in a public place with someone gabbing loudly, so we should all know how incredibly rude that is. Save your long, loud conversations for your car or your home—not a restaurant or Neiman Marcus! Ugh!

My rule is that anything I do on a computer, tablet, or smartphone (or around other people's computers, tablets, or smartphones) is essentially public. Here's the truth: If you or I do something wild and crazy anywhere, people can take photos or video of it and post those online—and probably will. I can't believe how particularly dumb people are being about nude photos. If you're going to take or send nude photos, crop your damn head! I mean, c'mon, we've all done stupid things, but you have to take care of yourself and make sure there's no photographic evidence that clearly identifies you!

Anything you post online is public. Period! I don't care about privacy settings; treat Facebook and Twitter like the giant bullhorn that social media is. If you're on the fence about what to broadcast online, keep it to yourself. Less is more when it comes to status updates and tweets, because an air of mystery about your personality, whereabouts, and lifestyle is always more chic than oversharing any of those details.

Though it may seem safer, e-mail is just as risky—and ultimately just as public. Whatever you write in an e-mail can be forwarded. That e-mail is not just meant for the person you sent it to, particularly if that person is even the slightest bit untrustworthy. I know firsthand of many friendships ruined by forwarded e-mails. If you want to talk to a friend in confidence, talk to that friend in person—not via e-mail, text, or chat. The same goes for resolving conflict, because e-mails, texts, and other digital messages don't have any tone and can come off more harsh or terse than they are meant to. I mean, sometimes even I use emoticons on e-mails to make sure my tone is interpreted correctly, and I'm a grown man! But I have to!

Another setting where practicing good etiquette will really pay off is at business functions and social situations related to work. Manners can make you stand out among your colleagues. The old maxim "Speak when spoken to" usually serves you well.

And finally, network sincerely! There's nothing worse than someone who just wants to get a business connection out of your conversation, or who uses odd tactics like repeating names over and over again. Seriously. I wish people would just mingle organically and let professional connections happen that way instead of trying to force it. After all, I'm much more likely to help someone I genuinely like than someone who I know or suspect is trying to use me for the successes in my career.

Whether it's in a professional or personal setting, you will always benefit from being respectful and considerate of everyone around you. It's basically what we were taught in elementary school: the Golden Rule. Treat everyone as you would like to be treated. It's really as simple as that. Emulate gracious, classy stars from the past like Grace Kelly, Audrey Hepburn, Lauren Bacall— the list could go on—and you will leave a lasting impression that you're not only glamorous but have class and manners to boot. ★

# RISING-STAR REMINDERS:

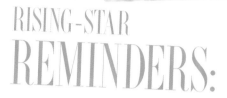

- ★ Be polite! Manners aren't just for Emily Post, your grandma, or fancy soirées—good behavior is as classy as Gucci and Givenchy.

- ★ The world doesn't revolve around you! Taking other people into consideration will be noticed and appreciated by others around you. It's a simple way to leave a significant, positive impression.

- ★ When you are introduced to people in a social setting—personal or business—it's better to say "It's nice to see you" if you're not sure whether you've met before.

- ★ Anything you do on a smartphone, tablet, computer, or camera—or anything you do around these devices—is *public*. Period.

- ★ Avoid gossip. It's déclassé, and it always, always comes back to bite you in the you-know-where. And certainly don't send a gossipy e-mail, because that e-mail can be forwarded to anyone!

# CONCLUSION

**Y**OUR INNER MOVIE STAR IS READY TO MAKE HER DEBUT. She has her closet of flattering outfits that suit her day-to-day lifestyle, with shoes and accessories to match. She has a great haircut, style, and color that match not only her facial features but her personality as well. Her powder room has a set of brushes, boxes, and jars ready to create a flawless beauty look. Her home décor is impeccable, and she can throw one hell of a party.

But more important, she has poise. She has confidence. She treats people with kindness and gratitude, never rudely or selfishly. She is a gracious guest, a generous host, and a polished colleague. She looks beautiful, put together, truly alive—and makes an effortlessly elegant, sophisticated impression.

As you've learned in this book, becoming your red-carpet-ready self is not achievable without some effort. But if you've incorporated my advice into your everyday life, you have also learned that exemplifying movie-star style is worth it. Being able to feel glamorous and luxurious—at any price point—is priceless. That's why I love fashion: It's not only fun and beautiful and luxurious, it has a truly transformative power for every single person who wants to experience it.

To supplement your hard work and your transformation from just someone to starlet, I'm going to share my tips on how to tweak your style as you age. No matter how old you are, you can look like a movie star. If you doubt me, take a look at Helen Mirren, Diane Keaton, or Maggie Smith. But as you grow older, you do need to learn a few tricks of the trade.

First, presentation is all about perception. Don't worry too much about "aging." I'm nearing the big fifty (well, in five years, but I need that time to mentally prepare!), and I'm perfectly fine and happy with my age. I have been for a long time. I don't even care about looking old.

That's not to say I don't care about aging, because I do. While I'm not dreading looking old, what scares the heck out of me is that I might end up feeling old, or worse yet, looking tired and fat. Everyone is going to look old eventually—but it's important to keep in mind that it's a choice whether or not to take care of ourselves as we age. It's never chic to feel old or look fat and tired—no matter how old you are. If I get more wrinkles on my face or begin going gray, that's totally fine! I mean, have you seen the other George? Clooney, that is. Being a silver fox can be sexy and chic.

But ultimately, having a few lines on your face or gray hairs is not a big deal It's natural to age, and it's chic to look your age. However, it's not OK to give up on glamorous just because you hit some weird age benchmark that exists in your mind.

A few years ago, I was in the running to be on a show that helped women look their age, and I was chomping at the bit because I love helping women look their best, whether they are fifty or twenty. Unfortunately, I didn't get that job. Boo. But fortunately for you, I still have a brain full of untapped advice on aging gracefully to share. They were fools not to give me that job, because I can make the average middle-aged man or woman look ten years younger in my sleep!

Whether you're thirty or eighty, you can look vibrant, youthful, and alive. Note that I say "youthful," not young. There's a big difference, and that's what most people get wrong when trying to look younger. Though you make yourself look younger at any age, many of us try to shave off too many years.

If you want to do it right, you essentially follow the same rules as before, just slightly amended for your age. For instance, it's key to keep flaunting your positives and minimizing your negatives. If you have great legs or sculpted arms, it's OK to show them off—at forty, fifty, or even sixty—so long as you cover the rest up. Give yourself a reality check every few years to make sure the positives are still the positives. Streamlining and simplifying your wardrobe as you age is smart, especially because you'll be shopping for and wearing more timeless, classic pieces instead of trendy fashions. The older we get, the wiser we are about choosing exactly what works for our bodies. We've tried a million trends, every style imaginable—and so we will know which might work and which never do.

The best way for an older woman to stay youthful and be up on trends is through accessories. While you may not be able to wear the clothes you see on the young starlets, you can still go out and buy that cool new shoe or handbag that's featured in fashion magazines, or don whatever fun jewelry trend is happening on the red carpet.

Another brilliant and incredibly subtle way to have fun with fashion is through nail art. You may think this sounds crazy, but my lovely cohost Joan Rivers always has fun, super-creative, and amazing nails. Whatever the kids are wearing, she's wearing on her hands. While Joan, and so many women even younger than her, may not be able to wear the same clothes as the new "It girl," she can incorporate the spirit and the fashion into her overall look. Joan is a woman who has never given up on taking care of her appearance or lost her zeal for life—making her a true star in my eyes!

Another way to maintain a flawless look is to make sure your makeup suits your skin, which changes as you age. Skin becomes less hydrated, meaning that the products you use—and how you apply them—should change with it. For example, crème foundations work better than powders on older women. In fact, any nonhydrating product will make skin look older than it is, by overemphasizing fine lines and wrinkles. In my opinion, less is more with makeup at any age, though you should never forget the transformative power of well-applied cosmetics. Your best weapon for keeping your skin healthy and young is proper cleansing, moisturizer use, and staying out of the sun (or wear sunblock if rays are unavoidable).

There are numerous stars who show us how to age gracefully. Women who look amazing at every age include of course, Helen, Maggie, Diane Keaton (who basically has been wearing the same wardrobe since ), Sharon Stone, Raquel

Welch (once a bombshell, always a bombshell!), Goldie Hawn (this woman looks happy in every single photo!), Halle Berry, Ann-Margret, Julianne Moore (seriously, she's fifty-plus?!?), Julia Roberts, Meryl Streep (so damn talented, who cares what she looks like!), Cate Blanchett, Geena Davis, Sigourney Weaver, Glenn Close, Susan Sarandon, and Michelle Pfeiffer.

# The Flip

THE TRUE KEY TO AGING GRACEFULLY is to look younger. Recently, I cleaned out a closet for a client in her early forties, and I was puzzled to find all these shapeless Nancy Reagan–type suits and separates. It made no sense to me why she would have these drab, outdated pieces in her wardrobe—until she told me that she wore them in her twenties and early thirties to look older. That's when I discovered the Flip. The Flip happens for most women at thirty-five. If you're younger than thirty-five, you are (mostly) trying to look older: more polished, more professional, more experienced, more sophisticated. But after thirty-five, the emphasis is to look younger. The mistake most women make, at that point and as they age, is trying to look twenty again (or God forbid, even younger). That's simply unrealistic, and it leads to dressing inappropriately.

At most, you should try to look five years younger than your current age. (Or five years older, if you happen to be under thirty!) If you are really lucky and have great skin (or have had good plastic surgery), you might be able to get away with shaving seven to ten years off. The key to the Flip is to remember: Before forty-five, go for five. If you're between thirty and forty-five, looking five years younger is achievable and reasonable. But after you reach forty-five, it's easier to shave more years off, though it's still safest to aim for five to six years younger. If you're forty, aim for thirty-three. If you're fifty, try to look forty to forty-five. At seventy, though, feel free to go for sixty. Beyond that, simply keeping up appearances will make you look good—and easily a decade or more younger than you are.

For my client, wearing those Nancy Reagan suits in her twenties worked to make her look more mature at society events. But if she wore those same pieces now, when she's in her early forties, she would look like she was modeling for the cover of . When I overhauled her closet, I ended up adding more tailored, sexy pieces because she still had a rockin' bod (why not flaunt it while you still can?), and tailored pieces would make her look more youthful. (Remember: When trying to look younger, aim for youthful, not for young. The saddest thing is a fifty-year-old woman trying to look twenty-five.)

Now that you share the secret of the Flip, use that knowledge wisely. It will not only help you avoid looking dated and old, but changing your wardrobe slightly as you age also helps you avoid falling into a style rut. Plus, it's an excuse to go shopping every year on your birthday!

The other key to aging gracefully is not about fashion. It's about having fun. Remember the Golden Girls? Those broads had more fun than most of my friends do! I actually hang out with the septuagenarian crowd sometimes, because we have fun together! Most of the time, I completely forget about our age difference, because every one of my older friends keeps up on current events and pop culture. Sometimes, I'll get curious and ask what it feels like to be seventy. Funny thing is, my friends say it feels the same as forty! And in their minds, that's not a bad thing.  And remember, a simple smile is the cheapest face lift!

My older friends are inspiring because they show how fashion and music can be a real fountain of youth. I'm not saying you should buy your grandma One Direction tickets, but keeping up with pop culture does tend to keep you up to date with society at large. At any age, if you're not current on pop culture, then you're not current in general. Talking about "the good old days" makes you seem old, whether the "days" were in 1950 or 1990. It's much, much more stylish to live in the present!

That doesn't mean you have to give up anything that isn't current. Many stars love vintage movies and older bands, like I do, while still being current. While a movie star wouldn't necessarily say that she thinks all music today is trash and that she loves the Beatles, she would say that she adores the Beatles and enjoys Rihanna. In terms of pop culture, balancing the vintage with today not only makes you great to have a conversation with at a party but can also help make you a well-rounded, sophisticated person.

No matter how much new music I listen to or how many pop culture trends I observe, in the end, I know I will get old. And though I may someday old, I promised myself a long time ago never to give up putting time and effort into my daily presentation.

I recently had lunch with my friend's mother, who is seventy-four. She was wearing gold shimmery eye shadow, a light berry lip color, and mascara—along with a great outfit—and she looked effortlessly glamorous. I bet she's put the same amount of effort into her appearance at every age throughout her life: at twenty, at thirty, at forty, at fifty, today. She has never stopped taking the time and making the effort to look good and feel confident before leaving her house—and I hope that this book has inspired you to take the same care and effort with yourself.

Now that you've captured the essence of movie-star style, there's no reason to step out of the spotlight for the rest of your life. ★

# ACKNOWLEDGMENTS

GLAMOUR IS DEFINITELY NOT EFFORTLESS, and neither is writing a book about how to look that way! I owe thanks to many people, including my agent, Peter Steinberg, for making this happen in the first place. My editor, Rebecca Kaplan, was helpful and enthusiastic through the entire publishing process, and Jennifer Levesque was a supporter from the start. I want to sincerely thank everyone at Abrams Image who turned my ideas into this beautiful book. And I have to thank my collaborator, the wonderfully fabulous Meghan Stevenson, who helped turn my many proclamations into the great advice you just read.

I'm also grateful to Art Streiber, who made *me* look like a movie star on the cover! But we also had help from Tibor Balazs, who hand-dyed the gorgeous Gaspar gloves just for me and Wendy Block, who agreed to let us shoot at her house and photograph her arms, (which conveniently came with a 12K diamond rock on her finger. Also, thanks to Torsten Witte for grooming my locks and powdering my nose.

In Hollywood, I have to thank Kent Belden and everyone at MMA for getting me here, as well as Brett Ruttenberg for sharing nice words about me. Ryan Haddon, there is so much more to come! I owe my start in fashion to Elizabeth Stewart, and in television to Cass Brownstein, who gave me my first hosting gig. I also want to sincerely thank Annie Roberts, who kept me on her casting list, and Kevin McClellan at E!, who took a chance on me. Without all of you, I wouldn't be here.

I also absolutely need to thank my truly glamorous cohosts Joan Rivers, Kelly Osbourne, and Giuliana Rancic, who keep me laughing on the set of *Fashion Police* week after week. These ladies make going to work a complete pleasure. I also want to sincerely thank every single person at E! (and beyond) who has had a hand in making our show such a success, including executive producers Melissa Rivers and Lisa Bacon, as well as producer Vanessa Katona, who takes time every week to talk about the looks we review on the show, and especially Ryan Randall, who makes me look good in every single episode.

My friends and family helped keep me sane while writing this book. Wendy Block is a dear friend (and "benefactor") when I most need it; William Holloway and Jean Louis Denoit helped me think beyond my world (and shared their world with me); and Magda Berliner was always there for me to talk shop when I needed to whine.

Last but not least, I simply would not have become the stylist I am today without watching my big sisters create their beauty looks during the 1980s, so I have to thank my family for that experience and millions more, all of which created who I am today. My brave sister Jean even agreed to let me share her waist-cincher transformation in this book! Thanks to my entire family. I may not get back to Illinois as much or as often as I would like, but I love you all very, very much. ★

# PHOTO CREDITS

Getty Images; **page 88:** (top left) Keystone-France/Gamma-Keystone via Getty Images; (top right) Steve Granitz/WireImage; (bottom left) Steve Granitz/WireImage; (bottom right) Silver Screen Collection/Getty Images; **page 89:** (top left) John Kobal Foundation/Getty Images; (top right) Ron Galella, Ltd./Getty Images; (bottom left) Time & Life Pictures/Getty Images; (bottom right) Hulton Archive/Getty Images; **page 90:** (top left) United Artist/Archive Photos/Getty Images; (top right) Ron Galella/WireImage; (bottom left) Willy Rizzo/Paris Match via Getty Images; (bottom right) Hulton Archive/Getty Images; **page 91:** Margaret Chute/Getty Images; **page 92:** John Kobal Foundation/Getty Images;

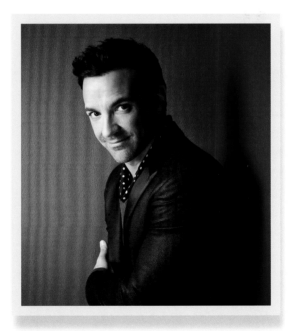

**page 95:** Columbia TriStar/ Getty Images; **page 97:** John Kobal Foundation/Getty Images; **page 98:** General Photographic Agency/Getty Images; **page 101:** Scotty Welbourne/John Kobal Foundation/Getty Images; **page 102:** John Kobal Foundation/ Getty Images; **page 105:** Photoshot/Getty Images; **page 108:** Ron Galella/WireImage; **page 110:** Ron Galella/WireImage; **page 115** Barry King/WireImage; **page 117:** John Kobal Foundation/Getty Images; **page 118:** Gilles Petard/ Redferns; **page 121:** Paramount Pictures/Courtesy of Getty Images; **page 128:** (top left) Terry O'Neill/Getty Images; (top right) Ron Galella/WireImage; (bottom left) Silver Screen Collection/Getty Images; (bottom right) Ron Galella/WireImage; **page 129:** Gilles Petard/Redferns; **page 135:** Gilles Petard/Redferns; **page 136:** Paramount Pictures/Getty Images; **page 151:** Paramount Pictures/Getty Images; **page 152:** Pictorial Parade/Hulton Archive/Getty Images; **page 158:** Alain BENAINOUS/Gamma-Rapho via/ Getty Images; **page 165:** Pictorial Parade/Hulton Archive/Getty Images

Editor: Rebecca Kaplan
Designer: Evan Gaffney
Production Manager: Anet Sirna-Bruder

Library of Congress Control Number: 2013935985

ISBN: 9781419706905

Text copyright © 2014 George Kotsiopoulos

Photo credits appear on pages 174–75.

Printed and bound in China
10 9 8 7 6 5 4 3 2 1

Abrams Image books are available at special discounts when purchased in quantity for premiums and promotions as well as fundraising or educational use. Special editions can also be created to specification. For details, contact specialsales@abramsbooks.com or the address below.

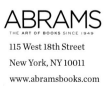

THE ART OF BOOKS SINCE 1949

115 West 18th Street
New York, NY 10011
www.abramsbooks.com